BASED ON THE FITNESS BLOG

# FOLLOWING
# FIT

MY ONGOING JOURNEY TO UNDERSTAND
ALL THINGS FITNESS AND NUTRITION

KRISTEN PERILLO

*For David, who lets me become.*

# *Forward*

I was once known as "the bread thief."

When I was a kid, it was always my job to slice the Italian bread for dinner. I'm not sure if this task was self-imposed, or if my parents assigned it to me, but everyone knew slicing bread was my jam.

Of course, the bread basket never really made it to the table as full as it should have been. One crusty end was already eaten by the time I sliced up half the loaf. And by the time I was finished slicing, another slice or two was inexplicably missing.

Once dinner was finally served, a good third of that loaf of bread was missing.

"The bread thief struck again," someone would snicker, reaching into the less-than-overflowing basket.

That's how much of my childhood passed. I loved carbs and hated meat so much I became a vegetarian in my 20s. And while I was healthy, for the most part, there was just one thing: I didn't move much. At all.

Up until my 30s, my few athletic endeavors were all failures.

I lost foot races when I was a kid. Running always made my sides hurt. I didn't like it. I struck out whenever I was at bat, so I skipped gym class every spring when we went outside for baseball games. And I tried to defend my brother from the neighborhood bully one day, but all I could think of to do was hit the kid with one of those over-sized, red, plastic wiffle ball bats.

The force of that bat was meek, like me.

Even the one somewhat athletic endeavor I had as a child—ballet—was a failure. When I was around 12 years old, my ballet peers were starting to move up to pointe classes. I'd been taking ballet since I was 3 or 4, and while I was never super enthusiastic about it, I thought I might want to give pointe a shot.

My teacher was a childhood friend of my father's. She told my parents I'd have to take extra classes, probably 2-3 per week, to get myself up to speed. Some of the girls were already in multiple classes, so I presumed this was to help me catch up.

One day in class, however, as we were practicing our positions, my teacher came over to correct my legs. As she helped me adjust my turnout, she touched my right leg, just above the knee, to guide it and said, "Us Italian girls with Italian thighs probably shouldn't be ballerinas anyway."

I was done with ballet after that. No pointe. No extra classes.

And thus my only foray into any kind of lasting physical achievement as a child ended when I was 12.

It wasn't until I was almost 32-years-old, after joining a gym with my brother, that I experienced any kind of impulse to be athletic. I had a few free sessions with a trainer, and after considering my history of incapability when it came to sports, I realized all of my prior accomplishments, as a student, a teacher, and a writer, had never been enough to make me feel fully comfortable in my skin.

I knew a lot of wonderful things about the world, about literature, and about life, but I lacked knowledge in a very important way:

*I didn't know shit about my body.*

And it was time to fix that.

I started lifting, and at first, I was a weakling, squatting just a 12-pound body bar. I did boot camp classes where I was the slowest person in the room. When our class went outside for the first time and had to run laps around the plaza, I walked most of the distance. I had to. I couldn't keep up.

But every small failure, like not being able to run a lap around a building, gave me a new goal. I started running a few times a week precisely because I sucked at it. I trained until I could squat real barbells, not rubber-coated aerobics class accessories. I matched my diet to my training goals.

And I found myself in love with my body for the first time—and not just because I liked how it was starting to look. I loved my body for what it was starting to do.

That epiphany spawned a series of life events that permanently changed who I am, and I chronicled many of those events on my blog, *Following Fit*. On *Following Fit*, I wrestled with my history as the "bread thief," with giving up vegetarianism, with my identity as a teacher, with returning to grad school for Nutrition, and eventually, with my own binge eating.

In 2018, after 8 years and over 600 posts, I shut *Following Fit* down. It was time to move on as a writer and move back to my writing roots—fiction, poetry, and narrative nonfiction.

But the original intent of *Following Fit*, captured in its subtitle—my ongoing journey to understand all things fitness and nutrition—lives on in everything I do, with or without a website.

What I thought was a journey to understand fitness and nutrition turned into a journey to understand myself. And that journey is, indeed, ongoing. No matter what I am, no matter what I become, that journey does not stop.

I am forever following fit.

*1*

The biggest failure I remember as a kid was Course 3 math, sophomore year of high school. And really, this wasn't a failure; I was good at math. Really good. I had the same math teacher for three straight years: Mr. Soffin. Throughout Courses 1 and 2, I was out for perfection, so much so I scored 100 on both the Course 1 and Course 2 exams. On the first day of Course 3, I told Mr. Soffin I was going for the three-peat. That was success in my eyes—the way to be successful was to make no mistakes, to achieve mathematical perfection. He simply nodded and said okay.

Of course, the exam rolled around in June, and I mistakenly inverted a parabola (or something) in the graphing section of the exam, and I wound up with a 97. When Mr. Soffin told me, I must've looked devastated, but he didn't say much except to tell me what I had done wrong. Instead, he called my house that night to talk to my mom. He wanted to make sure I was okay, to make sure I knew it didn't matter, and to say he was proud of what I'd done anyway. It may have been the only time a teacher ever called my house for something I had done.

That Course 3 exam typifies the attitude I had about failure for most of my life; failure, for me, wasn't about whether or not I could actually do something. It was always about whether or not I could do something well. Mediocrity was failure in my eyes, and I'd always had a hard time settling into the notion that average was acceptable.

So when I started strength training in June of 2009, I also started a boot camp class as part of my overall program. Boot camp is just what it sounds like—lots of cardio combined with body weight resistance. Push-ups, squats, lunges, stairs, running, jumping jacks, and the like. If you think someone might do it in basic training, we've probably done it in boot camp. On my first outdoor boot camp, we had to run a lap around the plaza in which the gym was located. I watched half the class pass me within seconds, turning the corner to go around the building before I'd even made it 30 yards. And then, halfway through the lap, I couldn't run anymore. I was out of breath, my chest was heaving, and my legs were pissed off. Failure? Utter and complete. For the first time I can remember in my life, this was not a failure to be the best. This was a failure to even be average.

I was angry. I didn't know at whom. It wasn't my body's fault I had never conditioned it to run. It wasn't my lungs' fault I had smoked for ten years, a pack a day, and that I still hadn't fully shaken some of the side effects even after having quit four years earlier. It wasn't even really *my* fault. Sure, I hadn't exercised regularly, and obviously, the smoking was of my own volition, but no one had ever taught me I should physically do things, that I should "work out" in some way. This was, in essence, my first attempt at running since I was a kid playing touch football in the street. Despite the irrationality of it, I was angry. I needed to fix this.

The easiest fix was to start running. I had no idea how hard that would be. I started on the treadmill, jogging at 5 mph, trying to keep the jog going for at least 8 to 10 minutes per session. When I was happy with my progress, I moved up my time and my speed. By July, I thought I was ready to start running outdoors. I think I made it through two weeks of regular morning runs before the tendon in my left ankle got sore. I had to take a few weeks off from running to my chagrin. But by September, I was up to 3 treadmill miles per session, averaging close to 6 mph. I wasn't fast, but I was running.

This was the first time I was confronted with my own mediocrity, but the experience is one I wouldn't change. I started to run intervals on Sundays—short slow jogs followed by intense sprints—because I wanted to make running, even on a treadmill, into something with which I could continue to challenge myself. One Sunday, I hit 6 miles of intervals in less than 60 minutes, a new personal benchmark. I know I am never going to be the best when it comes to running. I know people who run faster than I do, for longer distances, and in worse conditions than my safe little treadmill bubble. But I also know, without a doubt, if I hadn't failed so miserably at that first boot camp, I never would have challenged myself to add running to the list of fitness goals I was quickly accumulating. Failure, for me, has been a good thing. It pushes me to be better, and it's no longer "better" by the random numerical standards I imposed on myself in high school. Failure pushes me to be better by my own standards, and while my standards may still be high, they are personal, and those standards are the most fulfilling ones to achieve.

*2*

Once I really started paying attention to nutrition, I came to hate telling people how and what I was eating. Their faces told the story before they even opened their mouths to comment on my diet. Their eyes slid into disbelieving slits, sometimes their mouths pursed a little, their heads turned slightly away from me, and if their eyes wandered, it was to check and see what the rest of me looked like while I finished telling them tofu was not the food of the devil. And at least half of the people I spoke to followed up by asking, "Don't you like to eat?" or "Don't you have a vice?"

And the truth is, I do have a vice—peanut butter. I love it. I sometimes dream of it. I buy the natural, no preservatives, no sugar added, no salt added, no oil added stuff—ingredient: peanuts. Literally. And if I could, I would eat it from the jar every day, with a long-handled dessert spoon so I could get every last little bit of thick yumminess, every last little bit of crunchy peanut embedded within. I'd eat half the jar in one sitting, giant globs of it dripping from my elegant long spoon. Who'd care if my mouth was so dry from peanutty stickiness that I couldn't speak? Peanut butter's worth that kind of sacrifice, right?

But here's how I really eat it: half a tablespoon, in my oatmeal, with some cinnamon. Simple. No elegant long-handled spoon, no dry peanut mouth. And the difference between what I can envision myself doing and what I actually do speaks to my relationship with food pretty well. I love food. I love to eat. I love to cook. I buy cookbooks more often than novels. I read food blogs and nutrition websites more often than political news feeds. I watch cooking shows despite my vegetarianism and Food Network's carnivorism. I finish one meal and, shortly thereafter, start pondering my next. I like planning menus for parties, or dinners, or Saturday night snacks. I wander the grocery store with a cup of coffee because groceries are an event in my world. I linger in the bakery aisle. And I am always looking for a new restaurant to feed the obsession.

But what most defines my relationship with food is just what it seems like I might lack—control. I don't over-anything when it comes to food: overstuff, overindulge, overcook, nothing. I eat what I should, I eat what is appropriate, I eat what fills me, and I enjoy every last bit. We assume, in our culture, that loving and appreciating food means we must lack self-control, we must repeatedly show our love by overeating, or we must find emotional comfort in food. I do these things sometimes, too. But maybe the exact opposite is what we should strive for—maybe loving and appreciating food doesn't mean attaching an emotional value to it. Maybe it doesn't mean stuffing ourselves until our bodies punish us with heartburn and indigestion and our brains punish us with guilt and resolutions to try harder to resist. Maybe loving food is about treating it as we would our human loved ones—with respect and honor, not smothering and suffocation. Maybe loving food is about loving it for what it is—sustenance, nourishment, necessity, fun, and art.

Or maybe loving food is about loving our bodies and ourselves—about being committed to loving ourselves by being committed to healthy foods. Even peanut butter can be healthy when it's not eaten in giant dripping globs from a long-handled dessert spoon.

*3*

I tell my Media Analysis students, in the first week of
class, the TV show that means the most to me, that best
represents how I came to be who I am today, is
*Roseanne*. Some of them don't even know what the show
was—having been born well after the 90s, many of them
haven't even seen *Roseanne* in reruns. But the show
typifies the life I had as a kid. My family did not have
lots of money. We struggled to make ends meet. My
father lost a steel plant job in the early 80s, and there
were no college funds or summer cottages in my world.

The family on *Roseanne* seemed so familiar to me—more
familiar than the families on concurrent shows like *Full
House*—right down to the couch in the living room. We
had the same brown and orange plaid couch as the family
on *Roseanne* for years, a manifestation of the blue-collar
issues so well-represented by that show.

The similarities of my upbringing and *Roseanne* don't
end at the couch, either. They continue right into the
kitchen. Further, right into the pantry, where breakfast,
lunch, and dinner were unapologetically blue-collar.
Some of the food staples of *Roseanne* and my childhood
will sound more "American" than "blue-collar" to most:
meatloaf, hot dogs, burgers, pizza, Sunday pot roast,
sloppy joes. And yes, plenty of middle-class families eat
these foods on a regular basis; these are not strictly blue-
collar fodder. But the rest of what's in my childhood
pantry is certainly based not only in an "American" way
of eating but on price and convenience. The blue-collar

family not only has to buy food that will successfully feed a family for less money; this family also has to buy food that can be made in a hurry, sometimes by the kids, because the parents work long, tiring hours and don't have the daily luxury of time to make even a "home-cooked" American meal.

That's where processed foods come in—cheap, easy to buy, quick to cook, and even kids can prep them. Meals in my childhood included many of the staples of the processed food industry: chicken patties, fish sticks, tater tots, frozen french fries, boxed mac & cheese, jarred pasta sauce, Captain Crunch, fruit roll-ups. Friday night dinner was often the ultimate in processed seafood dinners, Tuna Helper. Or, even better, tuna casserole, the recipe for which I still know very well—boxed mac and cheese, a can of cream of mushroom soup, a can of peas and carrots, a can of tuna. Serve over warmed white dinner rolls. Notice what's missing: green things. Vegetables, when we did eat them, were often corn, broccoli, or carrots, steamed on the side, clearly not the focus of the meal.

The real ugliness of my childhood food experience goes beyond dinner. It was what I ate outside my parents' jurisdiction.

School breakfasts were faster and cheaper than eating at home. Twenty-five cents, in high school, bought me two bowls of Lucky Charms, a plastic-wrapped cinnamon bun, milk, and apple juice. I didn't buy school lunches often. I didn't like the meat-type-stuff they served, and if

I could avoid meat, I would. Instead, I would spend the seventy-five cents I had to get snack foods. Lunch, all through middle school, was an ice cream novelty on a stick and a bag of Cheez-Its. And milk. I distinctly remember middle school as the years of the candy bar for me as well. I had a teacher who often sold candy bars to students, like Milky Ways and Reese's Peanut Butter Cups, and I think I spent half of the seventh grade buying these for lunch when I was tired of ice cream and Cheez-Its.

It wasn't all about school, either. We used to go to a free lunch program for neighborhood kids in the summer, where lunch was often bologna and cheese, ham and cheese, or slimy roast beef on cold white rolls. Mustard, ketchup, and mayo came in little packets, just like fast food. (These packets were great for collecting and throwing under the tires of passing semis on the walk home.)

Sandwiches usually came with fruit—an apple, a banana, an orange. Milk and juice (usually frozen) were also available. And on special days, the free lunch had a treat: fruit popsicles, ice cream sandwiches, pizza slices in odd little cardboard boxes, or somewhat frozen peanut butter and jelly sandwiches on graham-cracker-cookie bread. Even when we went to the local elementary school's summer day camp, where we could swim, play in the gym, or make crafts, lunch seemed to be from the same standard-issue government source.

Don't get me wrong. By calling my childhood life with food "blue-collar," I do not mean to denigrate the job my parents did raising and feeding us. Or anyone else, for that matter. We all do the best we can with the knowledge we have. Yes, I remember government cheese in my refrigerator. Yes, I remember no-name fast food burgers, maybe forty-nine cents each, that were so gross to me I would line the roll with potato chips (our side dish) so I could get them down before I knew what I was eating. And yes, I remember eating out at a neighborhood diner, where prices (even today) are dirt cheap, as a once in a while treat. My parents did what any other family in their financial position would have done; they fed us what we kids were willing to eat as best they knew how.

And there is another part of the picture. It wasn't just boxes of things all the time. My parents cooked, too. My mother made a delectable beef stew. Even when I didn't like to eat meat as a kid, I always ate her beef stew. Sunday dinners were often fully home-cooked, traditional comfort foods—roasts, chicken, turkey, mashed potatoes, homemade gravy, fresh veggies. The weeknights were about quickness, especially once my brother and I were old enough to cook for ourselves and had busy schedules and our own part-time jobs. In the end, this quickness and necessity are what define my childhood eating as "blue-collar."

Lots of middle-class American kids eat processed foods, school lunches, and fast food burgers. The food industry taught us well, after World War II, that this was how modern Americans eat, and as a country, we shifted from homemade, localized foods to industrialized, processed foods as we were asked. But the middle-class American family gets to choose to eat this way; blue-collar families don't have the luxury of that choice. Chicken patties are still cheaper than organic chicken breasts. Fast food burgers are still cheaper than lean, grass-fed beef and whole grain rolls. And Captain Crunch is still cheaper than whole-grain low-sugar cereals.

Saying my childhood life with food was "blue-collar" is simply about making the distinction between who is allowed in this country to eat nutritionally sound foods and who isn't. Blue-collar families cannot afford, in either time or money, anything other than what the traditional American diet and the processed food industry has given them. And if you've never been poor, you just don't know how bad that is.

## 4

I keep a picture of my husband David and me on the microwave in our kitchen, mostly because I like the frame, which a friend gave to me for a birthday many years ago. The picture is from sometime in the fall of 2001, and I don't even recognize myself in it. Everything about me looks huge—big hair, big glasses, bloated face, bloated belly. And that "hugeness" typifies my twenties. I wasn't overweight, so by "hugeness," I do not mean my actual size. Nor did I have an inflated sense of what my body looked like—I wasn't much heavier than I am right now, so by no means did I think I was "fat." By "hugeness," I mean my twenties were extravagant. When it came to diet and fitness, I ate and drank everything more than I should have and worked out less than I should have. My appearance in that 2001 picture reminds me of that.

Food and drink, in my twenties, was 90% enjoyment and 10% health. I thought I was eating relatively healthy foods most of the time, though my sense of "healthy" was really, as you'll see, about eating low-fat, high-sugar, low-fiber, low-protein meals that were probably not doing me any long-term good. It was, however, during my early twenties when I finally went entirely vegetarian, though that change didn't revamp my "healthfulness" as much as one might think.

Before going vegetarian, I was still eating chicken. I had given up red meat as a teenager. I would've given it up as a kid, but my parents worried I wouldn't get all the nutrition I needed if I did that. In fact, when I finally did give up red meat, I remember my mother asking the pediatrician if it was OK for a growing teenage girl to eat only chicken and turkey. Of course it's OK, if it's done correctly, and these days, there's lots of information out there for developing healthy and nutritious vegetarian diets for teenagers, too. Vegetarianism wasn't as widely popular back then, though, and there was no internet, so my parents didn't know, and they wanted to make sure they did what was best for me.

By my early 20s, even though I had given up all meat but chicken, I was definitely not eating well. I have distinct memories of chicken finger subs every Friday night. I worked at a local clothing store, and after getting paid on Fridays, I would often pick up a whole chicken finger sub, complete with all the typical toppings, hot sauce, and blue cheese dressing, to eat for dinner when I got home. I could down the whole sub on my own, and I often did.

In general, my diet improved when I did go vegetarian. But my daily staples were still not good choices. I ate mostly carbs all day: sugary cereals for breakfast; yogurt and granola for lunch; many pieces of raw fruit (sometimes five a day); bread for snacks; bags and bags of pretzels; and various types of pasta for dinner. I bought into the prevailing wisdom of the late 1990s and early 2000s—that low fat, high carb foods were the way to go. I paid no attention to fiber, protein, sugar, or calories. I cared about fat grams.

Some of the most overly processed, unhealthy foods I've ever eaten were things I regularly ate during my twenties. Some good examples:

An entire small DiGiorno frozen pizza for dinner. Sometimes I ate iceberg lettuce salad with it. Illusions of vegetables, I guess.

An entire package of Lipton Pasta side dish (glorified macaroni and cheese) for dinner, right out of the container in which I'd microwaved it. Nothing served with this—just pasta, pasta, pasta for dinner. Low-fat cookies for dessert. One word: Snackwells.

By the time 2001 rolled around, I was eating either restaurant meals or packaged, processed foods for dinner every night. David and I either went out or ordered food a few nights a week, and on the other nights, we would make packaged pasta, like ravioli, or an occasional homemade stir-fry. We were vegetarians, yes, but night after night of even vegetarian pizzas, calzones, Chinese and Thai takeout, and grocery store ravioli did not make us healthy eaters.

It wasn't until we got our first apartment in 2002 that we started changing our diets. Living together made us cook at home more often, so I gradually taught myself how to make more homemade dinners and snacks. We still ate processed foods quite a bit, but I was developing a growing love for cooking and reading about food that eventually would help change our diets for the better.

The turning point in that change was probably 2005, the year I finally quit smoking. I was 27, and I had been smoking for ten years. I was at a pack a day when I quit pretty much cold turkey in February 2005, though I had sometimes smoked 1.5 packs a day at various stressful intervals. Quitting smoking made me feel interested in my own health (imagine that!), and when I combined this with the growing interest in cooking I had been developing for a few years, I started to think more carefully about what David and I put in our bodies. I read more cookbooks, checked out vegetarian websites, and bought my first Moosewood book. I still made foods that were not "healthy"—I loved baking, for example, so we made lots of homemade muffins, spice cakes, cookies, and pizza doughs. But we were finally heading away from processed foods, a definite step in the right direction.

By the end of my 20s, David and I were cooking homemade meals more often than not. The new staples in our diets were varieties of whole wheat bread, pasta, and flours, along with organic tofu, fresh vegetables, homemade soups and stews, and fresh fruits. We still bought processed foods, but we tried to choose them more carefully. My morning cereal, for example, went from Cinnamon Toast Crunch and Special K Strawberry to Kashi Go Lean, a cereal David still eats to this day. My lunch, formerly often sugary yogurt with equally sugary granola and several pieces of fruit, became whole grain English muffins with cottage cheese, or homemade vegetable soup with sweet potatoes. By the end of my 20s, I started to become interested in fitness—another side effect of giving up smoking. I was doing lots of at-home workouts: yoga, Pilates, Indian dancing, and

DVRed TV workouts. I have a small collection of DVDs, still, that combine light cardio with yoga, Pilates, ballet, and hand weights.

By the end of my 20s, I no longer looked like the girl in the picture frame on my microwave. Even though I didn't set out to change in so many ways during those years, I do not miss the girl in that picture. And I have a feeling she'd rather be me, anyway.

*5*

By the year I turned 30, it was safe to say my food habits had changed drastically since I was 20. I spent a lot of days and weekends cooking over that summer. On Saturday nights, David and I would grocery shop then fire up the charcoal grill. We loved barbequed spicy tofu with pineapple and sweet potatoes. We often grilled portobello mushroom caps with fresh basil and bocconcini, eating them on whole grain rolls with tomato slices or organic ketchup. We always had salad in the house. I baked whole wheat muffins every Friday night, substituting yogurt for oil and butter, and flavoring them with pumpkin and spices, bananas and walnuts, fresh strawberries with vanilla, or chocolate with cinnamon and cloves. We made homemade pizzas, sometimes on the grill, with homemade whole wheat pizza dough, tons of fresh veggies, and low-fat cheese. We only ordered out once a week, sometimes ordering salads, and we bought much less packaged food than we used to.

My daily food choices continued like this until sometime in the fall of 2008, when, for some reason, I thought I was getting too many carbs and not enough protein. I don't know what spurred this. I think I had read that the USDA food pyramid guidelines that promoted 6-11 servings of whole grains per day were inaccurate and biased. At any rate, I modified things a bit. My diet started to look more like what it is today. A typical day, in 2008, might've been some Kashi Go Lean with fruit for breakfast, a Kashi granola bar snack, homemade high-protein vegetable stew for lunch with a banana and an

apple, some greek yogurt with nuts and a few whole grain
pretzels after school, and a large salad, topped with
veggies, and some kind of soy protein for dinner.

I gave myself "cheat meals" on Friday and Saturday
nights. We ordered out on Fridays, and on Saturdays, we
cooked a "moderate" cheat meal for ourselves. David
wasn't eating like I was, to be honest. Our diets were
diverging by this point, even though I still made his
lunches every Sunday for him. While I was letting my
homemade high-protein vegetable stew simmer on
Sunday afternoons, I was making curried tofu, cheese,
and vegetable pockets (kind of like a calzone) for David's
lunches.

Even though I had added some protein to my day, and
even though I had cut the carbs from my dinners, I was
hungry all the time. It was hard, for example, to come
home from school and only eat a handful of pretzels. I
wanted to eat half the bag. It was hard, too, at about 10
AM at school, to not eat three of the Kashi granola bars
in my desk instead of just one. And it was equally hard
on Friday nights to not eat four slices of the large
Circular Eggplant pizza we'd ordered from Pizza Plant.
Something still wasn't working for me.

In the meantime, I decided, with my brother, to join a
gym at the start of 2009. I'd never been a gym person.
My previously mentioned DVD collection and full DVR
was a clear indicator I worked out at home. But in
addition to knowing something wasn't right with my diet,
I knew I was getting as much as I could out of the home

workout routine, and I needed more. My brother showed me the inner workings of some of the weight machines. As it turns out, I found I actually liked the gym. I got a few free training sessions with my membership, and when I finally used them to really do some weight lifting, I realized I didn't just like the gym—I loved it. This was when I decided I was going all out fitness.

That decision is the one that finally changed my diet into what it is today. I switched to a high-protein, moderate carb, vegetable-loaded, no fruit, low-glycemic diet. That's a mouthful, right? In all actuality, this was a standard weight training diet, typical of what you might see in fitness magazines or on internet sites. Just like most weight-lifting diets promote, I ate at least 1 g of protein for every pound of body weight I carried. If I weighed 120, for example, I ate 120 grams of protein per day (spread throughout all meals, of course). I focused on complex, slow-digesting carbs from grains. No refined sugar or enriched flours. I ate piles and piles of vegetables. Piles. In one week, with just a little bit of help from David, I burned through 2 pounds of salad greens and 1 pound of baby spinach. And that doesn't include the other roasted and grilled veggies I ate on top of all those greens. I drank tons of water, at least a gallon per day. These are all standard muscle-building methods. I just happened to be vegetarian, too.

Despite how complicated that might sound, the only things I kept track of were grams of protein and grams of carbs. I didn't worry about calories or fat grams. Compared to the low-fat, high-carb diet I described from my 20s, I was eating more fat, fewer carbs, and more calories, and I was definitely happier and healthier for it.

It wasn't long before I saw the benefits of this way of eating and working out. Before I started eating this way, I always felt overworked and exhausted. Friday nights would roll around, and I could count on being asleep on the couch by ten o'clock. Even if David and I hadn't eaten a huge meal that night, my Friday nights were a time to catch up on sleep a bit. I was still having issues waking up in the morning, too—a throwback to my smoking days—and despite my best efforts, I sometimes took naps after school or slept a little bit later than I wanted to on weekends.

Once I started working out and changed my diet, everything improved. I fell asleep more quickly at night, I woke up more easily in the morning, I didn't find myself passed out in the living room on Friday nights, and I was regularly up before 8:00 on weekends. These days, even if I stay up a little later than normal, I can't sleep past 6:30 very often. I never thought I had an internal clock, but apparently, it was hindered by my lifestyle choices.

There were other benefits to this diet as well. I no longer craved the "cheat" foods that I used to crave. I still ate and enjoyed sugar sometimes, that's true, but I didn't feel as drawn to it as I used to. In fact, I still love it, as evidenced by some of the desserts I have eaten. But I didn't get mid-afternoon sugar cravings, and I didn't get late night sugar cravings. Day to day stress no longer made me want to eat. I suppose having a daily workout to release energy helped this too, but especially when it comes to changing one's body, there's some truth to the saying that results are 80% diet and 20% workouts.

For me, though, the best thing about eating this way was that it genuinely fit with some of the goals I was already trying to achieve before starting training. I was already giving up processed, packaged foods, and I was already trying to move toward whole food sources instead. I was already starting to make all my own foods at home as well—as much as possible, I wanted my foods to come from my own hands, not a processing plant. And my new fitness goals did not interfere with these food goals at all. Eating this way not only matched my political and social beliefs, but it also matched and benefitted my health and fitness, and it is a lifestyle I can still commit to today.

*6*

Summer of 2010 was not easy. Nor was it an easy year, for that matter. It started fairly well. My mother was finishing treatment for breast cancer at the end of 2009, and it was a great relief to start 2010 knowing her chemo was finished and she was on track for full recovery.

By spring, however, several things were keeping me in a fairly constant state of self-evaluation. These were the kind of thoughts at the back of your brain that slowly creep up on you, sneak their way into your otherwise normal ruminations, and surface in ways you'd never expect.

In May, I was spending most of my car rides to and from school thinking about all the decisions I was trying to make, all the stressful events happening in my life, and when I got home at night, even after great workouts at the gym, I was having a hard time focusing on getting actual work accomplished. I was behind at home, I was behind at school, and I had what felt like major life decisions blooming. My focus was broken, for sure.

I was relieved when summer started, and I actually felt great during my first official week or so off. It was refreshing to sit around and think without chores, grading, or after school activities hanging over my head. After about a week, though, I remembered I was starting school again in the fall—as a student. I wanted a Nutrition degree, but I had a ton of prerequisites to finish.

I had to figure out how I was going to manage to take eight undergraduate courses over the next year while still teaching full-time and continuing my dedication to my workout schedule.

In addition, my 13-year old cat, Gurdi, was sick. She'd been sick all year. I knew, based on her medical issues over the last ten years, that she would eventually develop some kind of cancer. But in June, she was not eating well, was not moving well, and was not enjoying life as I hoped she would. We have a wonderful vet, and he was honest with us: she had an intestinal tumor, she probably didn't have much life left in her, and we could only hope the fluids, steroids, and meds we could give her would help her quality of life.

It helped. Gurdi did great all through the rest of June, and she was eating like a kitten, two full cans of food a day. But somewhere around the start of July, she slowed down again. By July 4th, she was back to where she'd been in June, and on July 7th, after trying another round of treatments, it was obvious we couldn't let her go on like that any longer. We lost her on July 7th—perhaps the hardest thing I've ever had to do.

Needless to say, the stress of that summer had gotten to me mentally and physically. I was spending too much time thinking and too much time negotiating every little decision. Instead of enjoying my new goals—going back to school in the fall, renewing my fitness efforts, learning new things about food—I stressed. And while I continued my fitness program despite the stress, I didn't see the gains I was used to because my body was telling my brain to stop.

One week I tried to do just that. I started by going for a massage, and then I spent the weekend doing little things around the house to make my home feel like it was in order. That always helps.

I spent the first few days of that week doing some extra reading as well, partly to satisfy my summer reading goals, but partly to keep my mind focused on positive things. And I made extra efforts to keep my food clean and interesting since I always feel better when I am eating better. Not that I wasn't eating well before this, but I cut back on things I was eating too much of (cottage cheese) and increased the variety in my daily meals a little.

The changes were small but effective at that point, and I felt a little more motivated every time I went to the gym. I also had constant new ideas for food creeping into my thoughts instead of stressful worries. My body took to the changes well, too. My legs felt light on the treadmill again, my head felt clear, and I started to see the quick muscle changes I am used to in my body.

Despite my normal dedication, I do lose my motivation sometimes. It's not usually failure that triggers the loss of motivation for me, though; it's life. Sometimes it gets inside your head. And it's important to keep that in mind since, more often than not, we only see a small part of someone else's life.

7

In 2010, I couldn't stop thinking about my mother's breasts. I know that's odd. She had just kicked breast cancer, so it's not as weird as it may seem. But even then, twelve months since her confirmed diagnosis, I couldn't stop thinking of her breasts. She'd had a lumpectomy, radiation treatments, and four months of chemo. She lost her hair, her eyelashes, her eyebrows, and her appetite, and all I was able to think of was her breasts.

Strangely enough, I never thought of breasts as something that might connect us—or separate us. I was jealous of hers as a kid. I honestly never wanted to look like my mom—that is not an insult, believe me. My mother has beautiful light skin, blue eyes, strawberry blonde hair, and freckles. I just always seemed to take after my father anyway. I have his curly hair, his thick eyebrows, his cheekbones, his jawline, even his chin. My mom (and her whole side of the family) doesn't have a chin. At the point where her jaw ends and her neck begins, her skin slopes ever so slightly so that, really, neck and face seem one continuous line. No chin. Though I could appreciate my mother's paleness, blue eyes, freckles, and chinless face, I really was only jealous of her breasts. I remember asking her, as a teenager, how it could be that every woman on both sides of our family had "womanly" figures that I lacked.

Her response confirmed for me the envy I felt—she said she'd always hoped I'd be "blessed" with the same womanly figure she'd been granted. I definitely wasn't blessed. Still haven't been. And I've always counted my lack of womanly greatness as just one more thing that separates my mother from me—like being vegetarian or denying Catholicism, our breast differences marked our ultimate distance.

After her diagnosis of breast cancer, however, I questioned the actual breadth of that distance. Are our bodies, our breasts, really more similar than I'd always believed? Is the estrogen in her body any more potent a carcinogen than the estrogen in mine? How awful is it that the very chemicals that make us women—that biologically define our bodies, social statuses, and lives—can also cause us to be sick, impaired, and abnormal? And will I, like my mother, find a lump in my left breast at age 61? Is breast cancer the inheritance, the genetic stamp, that my mother will finally give to me? Or will our breasts, like our hair, eyes, chins, and all our other discrepancies, keep us separated yet?

I was still thinking about these possibilities when I talked to my mother on the phone one weekend. She was recapping all the recent "anniversaries" she'd experienced—one year since she found the lump on a business trip, one year since she told my father what she'd found, one year since the mammogram, one year since the biopsy, one year since she saw the breast specialist. She knew what she'd felt, where she'd been, what she'd seen, and what she'd heard throughout the entire process. She had more anniversaries coming up as well—one year since her surgery, where we talked her through a nervous pre-op, perhaps the only time I've ever seen her scared. One year since radiation, which seemed to take all summer, not knowing if chemo was around the next corner. And one year since chemo was finally prescribed and words like nausea, hair loss, and hats became everyday vocabulary.

As I listened to her talk about it, it still seemed so surreal in my mind. How had she gotten herself through this? Even the word "biopsy" would make me shiver a little with fear. And as she continued to recall for me many of the little details of her journey through and beyond breast cancer, I realized there could be one thing I might want to inherit from her after all—her strength. Who needs "womanly" breasts if you can have your mother's strength?

## *8*

It's the times of adversity that make most people back off from fitness. Keeping myself motivated isn't something I usually have an issue with, and I've spent a lot of time thinking about why. So many people have great fitness and nutrition goals, and they set out to meet them with the highest of hopes, only to find, two or three weeks later, that they've fallen back into old habits, old routines, and old excuses. How have I managed not to let the usual suspects worm their way into my progress?

Part of the answer is simple—I am the kind of person for whom failure is not an option, as I've discussed before. But the rest of the answer is about my habits—I love routine. I like regularity in my life, I thrive on habit, and I'm beginning to think this is the bulk of what keeps me motivated every day.

This love of routine, however, used to be the cause of many of my most unhealthy behaviors. It's actually a simple concept. Regular behaviors become habits, right? There's a danger, then, in beginning unhealthy behaviors, like smoking even just on Friday nights, drinking two beers every night, or bringing home donuts every Sunday morning. And those kinds of unhealthy routines used to be a big part of my life. For sure, one reason smoking appealed to me so very much was the routine of it. When I quit, the hardest part was not just the physical withdrawal. The hardest part was the mental readjustment I had to make at every routine moment of my life. Waking up in the morning meant a cigarette with coffee, and I had to create a new routine to replace the one I had relied on for so long. Leaving school every day meant lighting up at a particular moment in my commute, and for a few weeks after I quit, that moment in my commute was a tough one. Even my first Christmas after quitting, it was challenging to go to my mother's house on Christmas Eve and not go out on the porch for a cigarette after dinner. My unhealthy routines extended beyond smoking, too, of course, but smoking is the epitome of my dependence on habit and routine and how very terrible that dependence can be.

These days I am still dependent on routines, but I have converted most of them to routines that promote my health, fitness, and happiness in better ways. I work out on the same days most weeks, at around the same time each day, and I stay after weight lifting to do a similar amount of cardio after every session. I sign up for boot camp classes that run at the same time every week. I even have routines for food—I wake up at a certain time most days, eat at certain times on most days, eat certain foods at certain times most days, and drink certain fluids at certain times most days. Even when I change my routine, such as when I decided to try out fasted morning cardio, I quickly developed a new morning routine: up at 6-ish, feed cats, take supplements, throw on gym clothes, drink coffee, make coffee to go, step out the door at 6:45-ish, return home by 7:45-ish, get changed, make the bed, make breakfast, eat at 8:15-ish. Boring? Maybe. But I thrive on that kind of habit, that kind of ritual, so for me, it's not boring. It's reliable, it's reassuring, and it somehow makes me feel confident, happy, and invigorated.

The same is often true of the other pleasures I take in life. I love my Friday nights, for example, because I spend the afternoon after school just hanging out with David. We get dinner together, and I spend the rest of the night vegging with some TV. Sure, I sometimes do something else on a Friday night. But I always look forward to the routine Fridays, the ones where I do the same thing I did last week. The same is true of my Saturday mornings. When boot camp is in session, I get up early, eat, go grocery shopping or to the farmers market, have a snack, and head to boot camp. Knowing, when I wake up in the morning, that I have a plan makes me likely to follow it, especially when it is a plan I have followed several times already.

It might be deemed uninteresting to people who thrive on constant change, but for me, the routine has been a key factor in getting me where I am now. It's not that I am unwilling to change, because I am always willing to adjust my habits when I know they need tweaking. If I have to change something, I do, and I find a way to work the change into a routine that I can live with. In the end, for me, the routine is not unimaginative or boring. It is helpful and satisfying. It makes me feel accomplished, like I'm not just doing chores and checking them off a list, but like I am slowly crossing off all the small steps that lead to the big goals, the long-term goals, the ones that got me motivated to start those routines in the first place. And coming back to those routines in times of chaos can be comforting.

## 9

One time, she was jogging on a treadmill.

A few days later, she was on the stair stepper.

And another time, she was not only on the treadmill, but she was also on the stair stepper next to me, then she was on an upright bike, and then she was in the weights, doing leg extensions.

She's just another woman I'd seen at the gym, with one significant difference: she was at least 80 years old.

I'm no pro at guessing ages so I could be wrong, but she must have been over 75 years old. Her hair was visibly thinning, her face was pouchy, and she clearly had osteoporosis. 80 years old seems like a safe guess to me. And while there's nothing unusual about seeing older people in the gym, the difference is this woman was doing difficult work. She was jogging, not walking at 2.5 mph while watching *Oprah*. She was on the stair stepper, not idly pedaling a recumbent bike while chatting on a cell phone. And she was lifting weights.

I used to spend a lot of time watching other gym goers when I did cardio. I don't think that's unusual. I saw people watching me all the time, checking out how fast I was going, how much time I'd put in, what resistance level I was working on. That's human. During longer cardio sessions, I had even more time to really see what the people around me were doing. And most of the women over 50 in my gym did the same easy work—walking, biking, occasional elliptical, sometimes some bicep curls. These women thought they were doing what was best for them regarding weight maintenance and cardiovascular health. After all, we've been told for years that 30 minutes of activity, even walking, can improve our cardiovascular and long-term health. While this may be true, more evidence has shown that moderate activity is not enough to stave off long-term weight gain, and more vigorous activity is required to avoid the extra pounds that come with aging.

Seeing the 80-year-old lady in my gym reminded me of why fitness and nutrition aren't merely passing fads for me—these are lifestyle decisions that will change the way I live my life for years to come. I remember being a kid and thinking that I was going to be really old in the year 2000, the year I turned 23. I couldn't imagine myself being that old, yet somehow, in 2010, at age 33, I felt better than I did when I actually turned 23. Nowadays, I'm thinking about what I'll be like when I'm 83. I want to be independent, strong, and capable at 83. And while I hope not to have osteoporosis, I do hope to be like the 80-year-old lady in my gym—still lifting weights, still working out, and most importantly, still working hard.

## *10*

"Just don't overdo it."

I heard that a lot when I first started training. And I hated it. It made me angry. The warning usually came from people who weren't athletes themselves, so it annoyed me that people with little experience in this area felt compelled to school me on the "dangers." I knew, logically, the people who said things like this were simply expressing genuine concern and that, even if that concern stemmed from a lack of knowledge about fitness, the sentiment itself was honest and not intended to be hurtful. Nonetheless, I was annoyed whenever someone told me this. After all, this kind of warning presumes that I don't know my own body, that I would let goals overtake whether or not I felt healthy, and that I would allow myself to work beyond my ability to recover successfully.

Of course, it is possible to overtrain. I saw a story on a news show once about a woman with a compulsive exercise disorder (also called anorexia athletica) who was addicted to exercise. She was plagued by feelings of guilt and unhappiness if she didn't fulfill her self-imposed exercise obligations—obligations that were not normal, like three hours of cardio each day (with no athletic purpose like marathon training). This kind of obsessive behavior clearly shows that, yes, it is possible to cross a line from healthy (but more than moderate) exercise to an unhealthy addiction.

For many people, the idea of going beyond what is considered "moderate" is an automatic signal of a problem. We're very leery of anyone who is not a professional athlete who trains beyond "average" expectations. This fear is compounded when the person in question is a woman; the strong association between women and eating disorders leads many people to presume that women who train harder than average must have a problem. We don't make the same assumptions about men. Men who train hard might be called lots of other things—like meatheads—because of their assumed focus on the size and shape of their bodies, but men are not accused of having a disorder as a result of their training focus. This is, unfortunately, a gendered issue.

I don't mean to diminish the problem we have with eating and body image in this country. Eating disorders and exercise disorders are real things, and real women are suffering from them. But not all women who train hard have problems, and plenty of women in the world know how to balance hard work in the gym with truly healthy and satisfying relationships with food. Unfortunately, we still have women caught in a Catch-22 of sorts—either we're not skinny enough compared to the media role models with which we're presented, or we're anorexic when we work hard or eat healthy food.

The signs of overtraining are pretty simple—not sleeping well, constant fatigue, unusual soreness, loss of performance, lack of motivation. By staying in tune with my body and my mental state, I can pretty accurately tell when I am pushing too hard. If I suddenly dread going to the gym, something is wrong. If I attempt to do cardio that was, just recently, invigorating for me and suddenly find it taxing and mentally torturous, something is wrong. If I wake up too often in the middle of the night, something's not right.

I try hard, however, to never let my training get to that point. Someone asked me, not too long ago, if I was worried about overtraining. And in terms of weight lifting, the answer is no. I know that I allow myself plenty of recovery time, and I never feel compelled to do things that will either injure me or damage my progress. In terms of cardio, I work hard to make sure I am doing work I continue to enjoy and that doesn't detract from my motivation. I push myself harder than most people do, I know, but having an awareness of my emotional and mental health helps me keep my hard physical work in line with my mental needs. I've changed my cardio routine over the years, for example, moving away from long cardio sessions at night. I used to enjoy long cardio sessions; right now, short and intense is better for me mentally. This change has inadvertently pushed me to do more work in shorter amounts of time, and the new challenge to see what I can get done in 25-30 minutes instead of 60 has given me the motivation that I didn't know I needed. And on days when I rest or on days when I only do a short workout, I don't feel at all guilty about the time I'm not spending in the gym. The rest makes me happy to start all over again on Monday, and if I'm not happy to do cardio at an ungodly hour on a Monday morning, I shouldn't be doing cardio at an ungodly hour on a Monday morning.

And ultimately, that's the point—working the way I do makes me happy, not miserable. Taking time off to rest makes me happy, not miserable. Being aware of the source and nutritional content of the food I eat makes me happy, too. If I ever find myself thinking that these things no longer make me happy, I'll change them. It's never, in the long run, just about physical fitness. It's about maintaining and developing a self-awareness that reaches into every area of my life, and that's too precious to me to lose it by "overdoing it."

*11*

My parents have been married for 48 years. That's almost a half century. For their 40th anniversary, my brother and I threw them a party to celebrate, and ever since then, I've been thinking about what kinds of things their dedication to their marriage has contributed to who I am today. Something must've rubbed off along the way, right?

I think so. But I don't think it was conscious on their part—that is, I don't think they ever sat down and decided they needed to teach my brother and me how to remain focused on a long-term goal despite hardships. That lesson, however, how to remain dedicated to something valuable, is just what I think their marriage has taught me.

Over the course of those 48 years, there were plenty of hardships that could have swayed their motivation as partners and parents. There were job changes, job losses, moves to new houses, car problems, school troubles, fighting kids, misbehaving dogs, family politics, house repairs, lost family members, health problems, and cancer. Plenty of reason to lose sight of the dedication it takes to hold a marriage and family together.

More importantly, though, there were the other things— holidays, family vacations, Sunday football games, school plays, youth hockey, job promotions, graduations, inside jokes, birthdays—to help keep the commitment to one another alive and well. And there were victories, too, like successfully overcoming cancer, that only add to all the reasons to celebrate these last 48 years.

My parents never pushed me to achieve my goals, nor did they ever lecture me about dedication and perseverance. They didn't have to. I was self-motivated enough, even as a kid. But I don't think they realized how much of that motivation is likely to have been derived from them. My goals may never have been (and may never be) the same as theirs—I'm not a marriage and family kind of girl. And my mother often asks what turnip truck I fell off of because we always seem so vastly different in our thinking. Even with our differences, how could I watch their daily struggles and successes and *not* learn long-term dedication from that example? This may be the most unintentional lesson they've ever taught me, but it's probably the most important. And that kind of unintentional teaching is the best kind—the kind that stays with us the longest.

# *12*

I've been thinking about one of my favorite quotes from Lao-Tzu: "He who knows others is clever; he who knows himself is enlightened." I have always tried to conquer the mystery of myself, and until recently, I thought I had a pretty good system worked out. I'm an analyst. I reflect upon, deconstruct, tear apart, and rebuild every decision I make. Every choice, opinion, sentence, and turn is a careful representation of what I know of myself so far. I thought I was living up to Lao-Tzu's words. I applied my habit of careful reflection in every aspect of my life— emotional, psychological, and spiritual. I've even reflected on this habit of reflection: do I think too much? Too little? Just enough? Regardless, I always knew, with some certainty, that no matter how much I changed or experienced new things, I had the self-awareness to deal with anything that could come my way, always thinking about who I was and who I might become.

Until one April, in 2009, when shortly after joining a gym, I decided to stay on the elliptical for 45 minutes. I felt great. I'd never stayed on any cardio equipment that long. My elation over this minor achievement, however, lasted exactly two hours, until exhaustion and soreness kicked in, and I found myself prostrate on the couch. I had felt so strong when really, I was actually very weak. I felt defeated.

Nothing, until that moment, had ever made me feel less in touch with who I physically was. I'd always been an inadequate athlete, but that never bothered me before. I filled that inadequacy with other self-imposed challenges—academics, music, financial independence, writing, self-reflection. That moment, however, when I sat exhausted on my couch and reflected on my weakness, made me realize that, despite my efforts to know myself well as Lao-Tzu instructed, there was one aspect of my being I had neglected to truly know: my body. My physical body was, for the most part, a mystery to me, even after having lived in it for those 32 years.

Shortly after that, after a long conversation about women and body image, a friend mentioned that she had found that, after having a child, she could no longer justify being concerned with things like diet or fitness. She had something more important to think about—a daughter. She assumed a woman's efforts towards knowing her body were superficial, the goal being to look or feel a certain way as defined by men, society, or other women. And at first, her convictions made me feel guilty. I'd just hired a personal trainer, adjusted my diet, and started working out regularly. Maybe I was that superficial woman who should have been focusing my energy into more "worthwhile" pursuits.

Later, though, I had a moment of certainty about this. On the treadmill, of course. I was pushing myself to run five minutes longer than I had the day before, and I could feel my lungs closing up on me. To get myself through it, I took a deep breath and relaxed my ribcage as much as I could. To my surprise, my lungs opened as I exhaled, the tightness around my ribs loosened, and I smiled as I felt my body agree to five more minutes. I finally felt like my mind and my body had a connection, something tangible that tied them together, something I could quantify. This was definitely not superficial. This was as "worthwhile" a pursuit as one could get. I felt like I was starting to understand yet another aspect of myself, my physical self. I was coming one step closer to Lao-Tzu's ideal, and it made me think this is what life is really for—a series of mysteries on which to hone how I understand myself.

## *13*

Shortly after my revelation that being in touch with my body was just as worthwhile as being in touch with the rest of myself, I found more reason to think fitness wasn't just a superficial pursuit.

It happened because I wore shorts to the gym one February day in 2011. In Buffalo. This is what we Buffalonians do—as soon as the temperature hits 40-degrees, we break out the summer clothes. I was planning on running some intervals that day, and since most of my gym pants like to fall down when I run, I was happy it was warm enough to wear shorts instead.

Before I left the gym, I stopped in the gym's open stretching area to cool down and stretch out my legs (something I only do after running). As I bent over to stretch my hamstrings, I looked up into the gym's mirror to see my outer quads, just above my knees, were starting to look bigger. I could see the start of some muscle—vastus lateralis—making its first appearance. I even pinched it, just to see how it felt.

When I sat down and stretched my right leg out in front of me, something else caught my attention—a thin line, a "cut," running up my inner thigh. Hello, sartorius! I pinched that, too. Then I made my friend look at it, even though she was consumed in child's pose next to me. I even named it—sartorius—out loud, so she would know what she was looking at. And then that night, while getting changed, I flexed my right leg out to my side, just to make sure sartorius was still there. It was.

Later, when I was brushing my teeth to go to bed, I caught a glimpse of my right arm in the mirror when I reached forward to turn on the water. There it was—triceps, lateral head—and I thought I saw a bit of something else next to it. Long head? When I attempted to flex purposely, I lost sight of whatever had been there. This time I didn't pinch it. But I know what I saw.

These are the two areas, legs and triceps, where I saw less definition than I wanted to during my first year of training, where I felt like my hard work hadn't yet paid off. It wasn't that those areas weren't worked hard because, believe me, they were. But both of these areas took a while to develop for me—my legs turned leaner than I'd ever seen them, but I didn't have as much visible muscle there as I wanted. And my arms were really lean—they were the one obvious marker of my weight lifting during my first year of training. But I didn't have that singular sign of developed arms—the triceps horseshoe. And I still didn't have it after two years of training.

All this mirror-looking made me think about how long it had taken me to get to that point. I'd been lifting weights for over a year and a half. In most people's minds, that's a long time to work toward a fitness goal. Most folks want to see their results in six to eight weeks. And when they don't get to those results in that short period of time, they give up. Achieving athletic goals is much harder work than most people realize.

The time commitment it takes, however, is one of the things I love—a while ago on social media, someone asked the world what they love about weight lifting. I answered that I love the empowerment, but I also love the humility. It is humbling to think I am still not finished achieving my goals after all this time. It is humbling to think I am just now seeing a little tiny bit of the larger results I wish to see. It is humbling to think that, no matter how strong I get, there is always someone stronger, someone more experienced, than I am. And it is humbling to think that, no matter how much I can lift today, there is still more to lift tomorrow.

## *14*

Despite my reflectiveness, I'm a dumbass. Sometimes.

It all stems from my problems with "rest" days. I only
have two settings in my life—on and off. So I am either
working super hard (that'd be the "on" setting), or I am
doing absolutely as little as possible (that'd be "off"). I
don't really know what "active rest" is. I guess this is
when people do things like go for walks, or hikes, or
work in their gardens or whatever. I don't do those
things. Rest, for me, is the couch. With occasional trips to
the kitchen. Then back to the couch. In fact, I am resting
right now, and I will continue to do so until I officially
rest in bed later on.

This kind of approach to rest, though, causes me some
serious mental turmoil when I get too much of it. Lots of
rest, for example, makes me kind of squirrely. I have to
move—and I have to move a lot—or my brain gets antsy.
I get stressed. I get obsessive. And I need to channel that
energy into something fairly frenetic to relax.

So when I started gaining weight to try to add muscle in
2010, I was torn about cutting out my cardio. I was only
lifting four days a week. How could I rest for three entire
days? I tried it for about eight weeks, and by the end of a
few months, I was done resting. I couldn't do it. I needed
to move. So I worked some moderate cardio back into my
week. I needed to flip the switch to "on" after what I
thought was so much rest.

Adding moderate cardio back in hadn't been a detriment to my strength gains. Until it was, when I failed on one of my planned personal bests on bench press.

As soon as it happened, I was angry. I was so angry I kept repeating the same obscenities, loudly, until I realized the woman working out next to me could certainly hear my potty mouth. And I needed to get on with my sets, so I had to stop swearing at some point. Even now, though, I am swearing in my head. A bunch.

So how did I know that my failure was due to that cardio I added back in? I did some cardio the day before—stepper circuits with squats and push-ups. I did a lot of push-ups—75 of them. And what did I fail on that day? Yep, chest. Hence why I am a dumbass.

I know the solution here; it's relatively easy. Don't do circuits involving the upper body on the day before an upper body workout. Same for legs. So I'm not worried this will happen again. I just need a little time to get over the fact that it's my own fault.

## *15*

There's always that one person at the gym. The one who gives you pause every time you see her. In my case, it's the latex glove lady. You can never miss her. She even has a uniform. She wears the same outfit to the gym each time, and she sets up at each machine by spreading a full-sized beach towel over the seat, carefully arranging it so her clothing never comes in contact with any part of that machine. And then she sits down, rests for several minutes, and lifts—all the while wearing disposable latex gloves. The first few times I saw her, I was sure she was a nut job.

But one night, I left the gym wondering if she wasn't the only nut job there. What if I'm a nut job, too?

It started when I was doing squats earlier that night, ten sets of 10 for a total of 100 squats. My trainer was coaching a co-worker who was competing in a bodybuilding competition in a month or two, and in between sets of squats, we were discussing this co-worker's enthusiasm for this upcoming show. He wasn't just motivated and interested; he loved everything about what he was doing—the lifting, the posing, even the eating. My trainer said this guy was, genuinely, "mental." I laughed; it sure sounded like this was true.

Then my trainer turned to me and said I was mental, too.

"Really?" I laughed at first. "How?" I asked. "How am I mental? And about what?"

"This," he said. "All of this. You're mental about this."

"Really?"

Now I wasn't laughing as much. How was I mental about this?

"If you failed right now, on 99 reps, how would you feel?"

The truth? I would've been pissed.

That, according to him, means I'm mental. Then he asked me why I do this.

The truth? Because I love it.

His theory was that the people who come into the gym and start training and working out because they want to lose some weight, feel better, etc. are the people who are "healthy." The people who keep coming back to do what I am doing, who clearly aren't there just for their simple health, are the mental ones.

"Why," I asked, "are these people mental? Why aren't they champions?"

"They are," he said. "'Champion' is a euphemism for mental."

This entire conversation, of course, was mostly joking, but I thought about it repeatedly afterward. I thought about it all through my last sets that night. I thought about it even as I watched latex glove lady do her mini squats. I thought about it the next afternoon as I went to the gym in a snowstorm. I thought about it as I pulled four Tupperware containers, one blender cup, and a baggy of apples out of my gigantic lunch bag when I got to work. And I thought about it again when I was sitting in my car mixing a protein shake and taking my creatine.

And I came to a decision—I'm mental. And I'm cool with that.

## *16*

Somehow, I managed to make friends with several of the really old guys in my gym. I told David about both of them, and he immediately started referring to them as Mandelbaums—after the *Seinfeld* character.

One of the Mandelbaums went MIA from the gym once, and I didn't know why. I intended to ask about him, but I kept forgetting. Finally, after a few weeks, he was back, and I ran into him as I was putting my things in a locker and getting ready for my training session. It turns out, he'd dropped a 35# plate on his foot, and he had been home with several broken bones for a few weeks. That was just his 2nd day back at the gym.

As I was wishing him a good workout and starting to walk away, he stopped me and said he had a story I just had to hear.

"Yesterday was my first day back here," he said. "And when I was here, I said to Chris [my trainer], 'No Wonder Woman today?' He just said to me, 'Nope, not on Wednesdays.' Chris didn't even ask me who I meant—he knew it was you."

I remember laughing about this with him, but this wasn't the first time I'd heard this kind of epithet directed towards me. It reminded me of something that happened almost exactly a year before.

During the first week of May, the dog David and I had adopted just two weeks earlier escaped our yard. We spent hours driving around our neighborhood looking for Merle, our beagle, that night. We called the police department in our town and the neighboring towns. We drove around some more. And then finally, at around 11 PM, we spotted him on a corner just two blocks from our house. We chased him, calling his name, but Merle seemed to think we were playing some kind of game, and he excitedly ran away from us, tail wagging. We lost him in someone's yard, and two and a half hours later, we still hadn't found him again. We were defeated, cold, tired, and angry, and we went home.

At six o'clock the next morning, David's phone rang. It was our town police department. I didn't need to hear the conversation to know why they were calling—they'd found Merle on the local expressway. He'd been hit by a car.

The next few hours were blurry. The animal control officer came over with Merle's body so we could make sure it was him. We had to call our vet to make arrangements for his disposal. I had taken the day off from work when I knew I'd be out all night looking for him, and I spent part of the morning emailing colleagues and calling friends to let everyone know what happened. Later that day, I went to the gym for my normal Wednesday cardio session, and I went back to work the next day, hoping that getting out of my house would help me not think about Merle.

By Thursday, I thought I was handling it pretty well. I had my Thursday training session, I didn't bother telling my trainer what had happened, and Friday came and went in a blur. On Saturday night, however, four days of not dealing with the issue caught up to me, and I did something I never did—I ate to make myself feel better. Half a jar of peanut butter. And on Sunday, I still wasn't finished dealing with it. So I ate again, this time, half a small pie. Somewhere in between spoonfuls of peanut butter and chocolate cream pie, I'm pretty sure I bawled my eyes out. Come Monday, though, instead of feeling relieved, I was embarrassed. I hadn't put the peanut butter on my Saturday food log, and I sent it off by email to my trainer on Sunday, pretending everything was OK. When I got to the gym on Monday, I felt the need to spill my guts.

I knew, logically, I didn't need to be ashamed of the eating. It was out of character for me, yes, but the emotional reasons behind it were unusual and, I think, understandable. So I also knew my trainer wasn't going to lecture me. I was sure he'd just accept what'd happened and tell me we'd get back on track and keep moving forward. This is pretty much what he did, and I felt relieved to move on with my session after that.

But he must've sensed that I wasn't going to just "move on" that easily. And if that's what he was thinking, he was right. I push myself pretty hard, mentally and physically, and it doesn't go over well with me when I think I have let myself down. While I can't remember whether this happened during my session or if it was a follow-up text message, at some point that night, he said something to me that has stuck with me since then:

*You don't need to be superwoman all the time.*

As much, then, as it's amusing or even flattering for Mr. Mandelbaum to refer to me as "Wonder Woman," it also reminds me there's a downside to my approach to things. I don't always know when or how to cut myself some slack, and I am more comfortable being a rock all the time than admitting I have emotional weaknesses, soft spots, or insecurities. I like being the one who has it all together, the one who can seemingly handle anything. When I can't handle it, when I'm struggling not to lose it, I have a hard time admitting it.

I'd rather be too strong than too weak. But it would behoove me to try and find some balance—to be able to acknowledge my vulnerability at the appropriate times, to admit I have a kryptonite (other than peanut butter). Even Wonder Woman has an alter ego, right?

## *17*

David's 80-year-old stepfather used to have a little diet motto: "Whatever Kristen says."

That's not because I was qualified to tell him what to eat. Technically, I was not. I'm a high school English teacher, remember? And until I finished schooling for nutrition, I was not anything else. But David's stepfather had some medical issues that needed correcting—blood sugar issues, cholesterol issues, and high blood pressure. He dealt with all of them with doctor-prescribed medication, of course, but he was trying to manage these things with diet and exercise as well. So he ate oatmeal with oat bran and flaxseed every day. He stuck to lean meats and lots of seafood. He watched his sweets and ate fruit instead. He ate brown rice instead of white. He even ate Ezekiel bread, the low glycemic bread I told him about.

And we had conversations like this:

"Here's what I do," he'd tell me. "I go to the gym, and I get on the bike for a while. Then I stretch. Then I go to the weight machines, and I do this." (Bends his elbows, puts his hands by his shoulders, and pushes his hands forward, straightening his arms.)

"Yes," I'd say. "That's the machine chest press."

"Then I do this," he'd say. (Reaches his arms up above his head and pulls his hands down toward his shoulders.)

"Lat pulldown," I'd say. "Good. What else?"

"I do this," he'd say. (Lifts his legs up, so they're parallel to the floor, then bends his knees and lowers his legs back down again.)

"Is the padded bar on that one above your legs or below them?" I'd ask.

"Above," he'd say.

"Leg extensions, okay," I'd say.

"Then I go stretch some more," he'd say. "Then I do these for my arms." (Turns his inner arms out and bends his elbows, lifting his fists to his shoulders.)

"Preacher curl," I'd say.

"And these." (Turns his arms, so his fists face in, and straightens his arms in a downward motion.)

"Triceps, yep."

"So will all that help my golf swing, too?" he'd ask.

"Yes," I'd say. "But you should do the back of your legs, too. Try the machine for your legs where the padded bar goes below your calves and you push it down."

"Then I walk on the treadmill," he'd say. "Then I go home."

He did, and still does, this several days a week. He was never really overweight, but he lost a few pounds doing this. More importantly, though, I heard of other results from David's mother. His stepfather went to the doctor, and his blood pressure was so low his doctor said he might be able to stop his blood pressure medication if this keeps up. (This is, by the way, the same doctor who gave him zero guidance as to how to manage these health concerns in any way other than medication, hence why he often asked me if he should eat this or that.)

It makes me happy to see good results for a good effort. And if David's stepfather can do this, anyone can.

## *18*

When I first started lifting weights, people always asked me what my goals were. I think I spent all of my first year of weightlifting saying things like:

> *I want to be strong.*

> *I want to be athletic.*

> *I want to be fit.*

After a while, I got tired of those answers. So I started telling people I wanted to be able to bench press David.

David is something his friend calls a "Thin Tall." He's 6'2" and has legs that look like they go to his armpits. He's the kind of guy for whom gaining weight is difficult. Bench pressing him wouldn't be entirely out of reach for someone my size, but it'd take me years of lifting to get there.

Benching David, of course, has not happened. I can, however, say the following:

> *I can squat David.*

*I can stiff-leg deadlift David.*

*I can Romanian deadlift David.*

And I can also say:

*I can deadlift David, plus a 50-pound bag of cat food, off the floor.*

Just in case I ever need to.

## *19*

Saturday, February 26th, 2005. That was the day I quit smoking cigarettes. And I remember that day like it just happened.

Well, ok, I don't remember all of it. I don't remember, for example, my last cigarette. I'm sure I thought I was savoring it at the time, but I don't recall it at all. It must have been on that Friday, the 25th. And I must have smoked that cigarette at home, in the living room of the apartment David and I rented at the time. But all that isn't even a memory—that's me assuming what probably was the case.

What I do remember is getting up on Saturday, February 26th, 2005, and going to Rite-Aid where I bought some Nicorette. And I remember chewing a few pieces of that gum. It was kind of peppery tasting, and you were supposed to chew it and then wad it up against your gums to let the nicotine get in your body. Sounds appetizing, right?

I also remember that night. We went to my brother's house to watch hockey. I remember getting angry at David shortly after we got there. I remember throwing things, namely my purse, at David's head because I was pissed off. I missed his head, and my purse hit the wall of my brother's apartment instead. I remember my brother was pissed off at me because of this. And that's it. That's all I recall—I don't remember the hockey game, or eating snacks, or even driving home that night.

But I remember momentary smoking temptations after that: my first day back at school without cigarettes, my first ride home after school, my first Christmas without cigarettes, my first really emotional moment without cigarettes—when my boss of nearly 10 years, who had pretty much put me through grad school and student teaching, died of cancer. And I remember lots of milestones after that: my first realization food tasted better, my first realization I was losing my smoker's cough, my first attempts at working out without losing my stamina.

Today I don't celebrate this anniversary. On that anniversary, I'll gladly go to the gym, where I'll gladly do a zillion squats, lunges, push-ups, and mountain climbers, and I'll know, the entire time, I couldn't have done this kind of thing if I was still smoking. Or I'll go grocery shopping, where I'll buy lots of cottage cheese, egg whites, sweet potatoes, vegetables, and avocados. And I'll know, the entire time, that none of this healthy food would have made much difference in my body if I was still smoking. Or I'll watch hockey, maybe at my house this time, and while I won't throw things at anyone (I hope), I'll know, the entire time, that I can simply relax, enjoying the game and enjoying the company. For me, that's the way to celebrate this kind of anniversary— by doing all the things I couldn't when I smoked, and by doing them all with my health and my fitness in mind.

## *20*

My parents and the longevity of their marriage wasn't my only inspiration to be dedicated. I took some of my inspiration from my favorite TV show when I was a kid:

*The Incredible Hulk.*

I should have known back then I was a total nerd.

But I had a thing for 70s superheroes—I loved *Wonder Woman*, too. I even had her Underoos. If you're too young to understand that statement, google it.

*The Incredible Hulk* only ran from 1978-1982, and considering I was only five years old when the show ended, I must have been watching it in reruns. I specifically remember watching it with my friend, who lived two doors down, on Saturday afternoons.

I'm not sure why I loved it—I'd like to say my love for it had something to do with the idea of dual selves, some kind of natural attraction to the Jekyll-&-Hyde-esque characters. It is more likely, however, I just had a crush on Bill Bixby. And Lou Ferrigno.

For some reason, I had completely forgotten about my love for the Hulk until one day when my trainer gave me a copy of *Pumping Iron* to watch. *Pumping Iron* is, of course, the 1977 "docudrama" about the guys training for and competing in the 1975 Mr. Olympia and Mr. Universe competitions. The majority of the film focuses on the Olympia competition, with Arnold Schwarzenegger vying for his 6th consecutive title against both Lou Ferrigno and Franco Columbu. Despite the focus on Arnold, though, the best parts of this movie were the Lou Ferrigno sequences.

Like the scene where Lou is chanting Arnold's name while training.

And when he is learning how to pose.

My favorite Ferrigno moment, though, comes after the Olympia is over. The competitors are sitting around eating, singing "Happy Birthday" to Ferrigno. When someone calls on him to make a speech, his answer is simply, "I have nothing to say. I just wanna eat my cake."

I wouldn't necessarily recommend *Pumping Iron* to anyone who isn't interested in some of the history of bodybuilding. But Lou Ferrigno made me laugh out loud. And his statement to his father after losing the Olympia was inspiring:

"It will just give me the motivation to train harder."

True that, Lou.

## *21*

I will be the first person to admit most people cannot dedicate the time & energy to fitness I do. That's OK—I don't expect everyone to lift four days a week, take boot camp classes, and weigh, in advance, every morsel of food she plans to consume.

That doesn't mean "real" people can't be fit, too. It is entirely possible to be fit without all the craziness in which I partake. Being fit is about being dedicated, motivated, realistic, patient, and consistent.

Case in point: Danielle.

Danielle is my friend, colleague, and cardio buddy. In 2010, she gave birth to her first child. She quickly got back to her pre-pregnancy scale weight, and she ran her first 1/4 marathon at the end of May 2011.

Danielle was not in "bad" shape before she got pregnant; she was consistently going to the gym and continued to do so throughout her pregnancy, using weight machines and doing various cardio. However, she never really saw the kinds of results she wanted. She wasn't using free weights, and she wasn't training legs with weights. Leg training consisted of body weight work only, and the reliance on weight machines resulted in a strong upper body but a weak core. Her diet was low in protein, high in carbs—not earth-shatteringly unhealthy—but it was not helping her gain the lean muscle mass she wanted.

Danielle decided to change this, so she began a simple program—two days of full-body weight training, mostly based on free weights, including weighted leg work, and two days of cardio circuits with me. In between, she started running treadmill intervals when she could. When my trainer's boot camp class began, she signed up to do that instead of doing circuits with me. Shortly after that, she volunteered to not only run as part of a 4-woman marathon relay team but to run as an anchor—meaning 7+ miles. In addition, then, to her two weight days and two boot camp days per week, she was also training to meet her running goals in time for her Memorial Day race.

Danielle also changed her diet to reflect her new goals. Rather than relying on mostly fruits, vegetables and carbs, Danielle's diet relied on lean protein at every meal. Like me, Danielle was vegetarian, so lean protein often meant eggs, tofu, greek yogurt, cottage cheese, and whey protein. She was also dedicated to a whole foods diet—no packaged meals, no processed meat replacements—and as such, her carbs came mostly from whole grains, like oats, quinoa, and whole grain bread. She got healthy fats from egg yolks, peanut butter, nuts, and olive oil, and she loved vegetables with both lunch and dinner. She didn't track her food; she didn't weigh her vegetables. But for her lifestyle and her goals, her diet worked in terms of both foods that fit her schedule and her tastes.

Danielle is proof everyone can reach her fitness goals through the right workout and food choices—if those choices are accompanied by dedication and consistency. That doesn't mean reaching those goals will be easy. Danielle worked her butt off, and she knew the moment when most people would give up is precisely the moment when she must push herself even harder. But Danielle is also proof you need not be a bodybuilder, or unbalanced, to be fit. You must simply be persistent, and you must be willing to commit to hard work. Danielle shows that, despite the fact it isn't easy, it is doable, and it is precisely that hard work that makes it so rewarding in the end.

## *22*

Somehow, over the last few years, I wound up teaching half of my school's wrestling team. At first, I thought it was just my interest in weightlifting that made me notice who the wrestlers were. After all, I had been teaching at this co-ed high school for two years before I started lifting. Maybe I taught wrestlers then and just didn't realize it since words like "squat" and "traps" weren't yet part of my classroom vocabulary.

But after thinking about the kids I've taught at this school, I realized that I really had taught more of the wrestlers in the last few years than in any years prior.

This, in itself, isn't really all that interesting. What is interesting about it, though, is the degree to which I have found that I have developed stronger bonds with some of my male students precisely because of a common interest in weightlifting. And in general, it is the wrestlers who are concerned with things like squats and traps.

This new found connection to kids in my classroom has developed interesting, and sometimes silly, ramifications for my classroom activities. My favorites, so far, have been the ideas kids come up with when they hear about what I do in the gym.

When I broke my toe and badly bruised my foot, for example, after having a 25-pound dumbbell fall on my foot in the gym, I was out of school for three days. When I finally came back, my sophomores wanted to hear the whole story. Apparently, the boys (mostly the wrestlers) were making up theories about what had happened to me and why I was out three days in a row.

The best theory: I was squatting an obscene amount of weight, and it was so heavy that, while the barbell was on my back, I tipped over to the side, all the plates came crashing to the floor, and somehow, in the scuffle, I hurt my foot.

My first question upon hearing this was how much weight I was squatting in this hypothesis. The kid who made up the story pointed to another pretty strong boy in the room and said, "More than he can squat."

Then there's my shoulder—at 34 years old, I had arthritis in my AC joint, and it was interfering with my day-day-day activities. I told them I was a little nervous about having surgery since I'd never had surgery before. This lead to questions about how I managed to get arthritis in that shoulder to begin with. When I told them to take a wild guess what caused it, one boy yelled, "Squats, right?"

Once, while reading *Macbeth*, I had students work on an activity I heard about from a colleague several years ago—have students choose one of the four apparitions that appear to Macbeth in Act 4 and create a drawing of that apparition. It sounds elementary, but it is a fun break from Shakespearean analysis, and it seems to help students remember which apparitions are which.

The boys, of course, had fun with this assignment, creating overly bloody and gory apparitions.

According to some of the boys, Macbeth was visited by a bodybuilding apparition (if you know the play, this was supposed to be the crowned child holding the tree). When I held this picture up for everyone to see, they found it particularly funny this "crowned child" had not just some visible abs and pecs but rather large traps as well. Incidentally, I also found it amusing the apparition had some huge quads, especially since I've known several teen weightlifters who only do upper body. This ghost never skipped leg day.

There was even a day when I inadvertently schooled one of my students on creatine supplementation; he was doing a research project on the use of steroids in professional baseball, and I noticed that he had been taking notes on the effects of creatine in the body. When I mentioned that creatine was not, in fact, a steroid (though it was banned from baseball), he was a little dumbfounded. And when I then mentioned that I happen to take creatine, he turned bright red. I had to reassure him, again, that it wasn't actually a steroid, and his teacher was not going to grow a mustache, gain a deeper voice, or turn into a flaming ball of roid rage.

The fact that my students know about my interest in weightlifting has had a positive impact on my classroom. I've had some very interesting (and sometimes frustrating) conversations with students about things like the pressure to fit into a specific weight class—I had one student who, after not eating all day so he could make weight, was genuinely angry when after-school activities were canceled due to weather that day. "I could've had lunch," he said. And I've had many conversations with kids about proper form, about how much cardio one should do, and about why I love weightlifting in the first place.

These conversations, however, have made me lament the fact I've only been able to connect with male students on these terms—female high school athletes don't seem to hit the weight room often. I taught for four years at an all-girls school before moving to a public school, and even if I had been lifting back then, I don't think I would've been able to use that passion to help forge strong connections to girls. That's not to say there weren't great student-athletes at that school—some of the strongest female athletes I taught back then are still athletes today—and some of them used to read and comment on my blog.

Instead, I still find myself connecting with female students through the stereotypical "feminine" things—clothing, shoes, jewelry, a love for Johnny Depp. Even when I have the chance to talk fitness and food with female students, the subject is never weight lifting, muscle, or protein powders. It's about dieting, salad, or body image.

I am glad, despite their lack of interest, to have exposed my female students to a woman who does lift. I would be happier, though, if they were the ones drawing pictures of over-sized quads.

## 23

Once, after accosting me at the end of a workout to discuss some Wordsworth lines with which he had earlier regaled me, one of the Mandelbaums told me a story I found a little disturbing.

Knowing I'm a teacher, Mandelbaum had once asked me if I experienced many behavior issues in my classroom. I told him I hadn't, except in the cases of students who genuinely misbehaved in many classes. For the most part, I have good students. He found this interesting, as he has a friend who retired from a local school district, and this friend often complained his students' behavior was getting worse every year.

After our Wordsworth chat, Mr. Mandelbaum said he'd told his retired friend of my comments, specifically that I don't have many behavior issues in my classes, and his friend's very first response was a question: "Is she attractive?" he asked.

In the context of this conversation, I laughed. But in my mind, this question infuriated me. The implication is that a woman would garner more respect—in the classroom or in any setting in which a power hierarchy exists—if she were physically appealing. My lack of behavior problems, under this theory, is attributable not to my earned respect as a teacher or the kinds of relationships I have with kids but to my physical appearance.

I quickly got over how annoyed I was at this idea when I found I could easily provide evidence of otherwise "attractive" female teachers who did, in fact, have problems with student behaviors in their classrooms. But the whole idea of the importance of physical appearance got me thinking.

To what degree, for example, am I in this fitness thing because of physical appearance?

I started lifting because I wanted to be strong, literally, and I wanted a connection to my body that was based on what it could do rather than what it looked like. That connection is very appealing to me—I hesitate to say that the connection I have to my sense of body now is "spiritual," but I do feel my growing awareness of my body and its abilities is something akin to being enlightened. Or at least to becoming enlightened.

Despite my original (and ongoing) quest for that connection, I still find myself drawn to the ways in which my physical appearance is different because of this quest. I wrote something not long ago about finally accepting my body and no longer seeing flaws. Turning to fitness was a way to inadvertently work out those body issues. Even without body issues, though, I am still turning to my physical appearance for evidence of my diet progress. I look in the mirror for new muscle definition, for veins, for leanness I didn't see there before. I may not be seeing myself as flawed, but I am focused on appearances—on what I consider to be attractive—nonetheless.

For a while, I tried to figure out why I didn't feel at all superficial about this focus on appearance. At first, I thought it was just the nature of what I am trying to accomplish—when one's goal is body-related, appearance has to be part of the evidence one uses to indicate success. I'm sure this is why some people still look at bodybuilders and see nothing but a "superficial" focus on physicality instead of the athleticism it takes to get that physicality.

But there's more to this than the idea that it's just the nature of the beast. Taking ownership of one's physical appearance is actually a way to defy the normal expectations of attractiveness in women. Taking control of my body is powerful, especially when my goals for that body aren't in line with accepted ideas of beauty for women. It seems odd to me when women sex themselves up and then claim that they are empowering themselves through sexuality. It's not empowering if you're doing exactly what society says you should. But perhaps it is empowering, and not superficial, to reclaim one's body, to remake it in ways that indicate strength rather than submissiveness.

Maybe I'm assigning too much meaning to something that's insignificant. I prefer, however, to think I am a rebel. Or maybe "rebel" is just a great euphemism for "nut job." Whichever. At any rate, I am very focused on appearances right now, and for that, I make no apologies.

Despite being at ease with my own focus on appearance, I can't help but mourn the fact that our mainstream media is still so focused on a particularly weak female body.

And when I think of the poster child for that weak female body, who immediately comes to mind?

Gwyneth Paltrow.

There's nothing about Gwyneth Paltrow that doesn't irritate the crap out of me: mainstream publications calling her a "lifestyle guru", her promotion of a diet that is just plain imbalanced and unhealthy, her "trainer" who insists women should not lift more than 3 pounds, the fact that Oprah promoted said "trainer," even the "before & after" pictures on her poorly named GOOP website. All of it irks me. The kicker, for me, was the revelation that Paltrow, at only 37 years old, had osteopenia. It doesn't even matter to me whether that health issue stems from her diet or her "weight" training; the fact is that this woman, to whom many women are looking for fitness and dieting advice, is not fit to be giving such advice. Nor is she, for that matter, "fit."

Paltrow is the unofficial mascot for the kind of female body I want to defy—not that her kind of body is even achievable. Even if one did train with the Tracy Anderson method and workout for 2 hours a day, six days a week, doing glorified cardio and drinking kale juice all day.

I've not just been lamenting, however, the popularity of bodies like Paltrow's; I've also been grieving the criticism publicly directed at very famous women who did acquire some muscle. Cameron Diaz and Madonna both took a lot of flak for their muscular bodies, being called not "strong" nor "fit" but "manly." Clearly, we still lack the ability to describe a strong female body in a positive way.

I know there are media outlets that promote athletic women—*Muscle & Fitness*, *Oxygen*, etc.—and there are athletes out there, like Serena Williams, who espouse a muscular build in unapologetic ways. But the fact is that those views are not reflected in our mass media. So until *People* is saying nice things about muscular women, I will keep mourning this.

I know I am not the first person to write about this, nor am I necessarily saying anything new about the subject. But after recognizing that it's not only OK but productive to be focused so much on how my body looks, I couldn't help but feel sad, too, for all the women who will never have that same experience, whose focus on their bodies is not positive, not productive, and not based on anything more than a Gwyneth Paltrow sponsored pipe dream.

## *24*

Back in early 2011, I started experiencing mild aching, kind of a nagging pain, in my left shoulder. I even modified my chest & shoulder training for a few weeks to give that area a bit of a rest. When I broke my toe that April, I started sleeping on my right shoulder to accommodate my foot, and this also gave my left shoulder a good break. The nagging pain had pretty much subsided—until late May.

Somewhere between sleeping on that shoulder, heavily training chest, and heavily training shoulders, my nagging pain was back. One Saturday, my shoulder bothered me for most of the day after my morning boot camp class. The pain was not acute, and there was no one trigger for it. Instead, it just ached. Usually, the ache was minor—the kind of thing I would simply work through. Occasionally, the pain seemed to affect either my outer delts or my traps, but for the most part, the problem was just as I have already said—nagging.

I decided I needed to get this checked out if it was going to be persistent. I wanted to make sure I didn't have some sort of impingement, tendonitis, or rotator cuff issue. That area felt most painful, for example, during rotation-based exercises and cross-body (both front and back) exercises, so it wasn't out of the question that there could have been something more serious going on.

Fortunately, because I saw an awesome orthopedist for my foot, I already had a doctor to call upon, and his specialty happened to be shoulders. We did x-rays, he worked me through all the movement checks, and he easily pronounced it arthritis.

Good news—it was not a tendon or muscle issue. I could continue to work out, including lifting.

Bad news—the then-mild ache would not get better on its own. It would need treatment—and the options were NSAIDs (temporary help), cortisone injections (temporary but better than NSAIDs), and surgery (permanent).

I chose surgery. And then I promptly scheduled it for July.

This was a little scary for me because, other than wisdom teeth (a nightmare!), I have never had surgery. But I told the doctor what I wanted to do almost instantly, despite my fears, because he pretty much laid it out for me. No surgery would mean long-term problems, no matter how much weight I could lift, and the pain would slowly turn from mild and achy to downright debilitating. Surgery meant I could keep lifting. Indefinitely.

Luckily, this could be done arthroscopically, with only a few small incisions, and recovery time was a few days if that. When I asked about recovery, the doctor said I'd be sent home in a sling, but I could "throw it away" as soon as I wanted to. Because he was not repairing either a tendon or a muscle, and because the problem simply involved removing some of the bone in that area, I could

return to "normal activity" as soon as I felt
ready. Translation: when I felt I could handle the
soreness, I could return to normal activity. I would have
zero restrictions in his eyes during recovery.

The mild ache wasn't just affecting my sleep; my form
was compromised, too. My trainer noticed my left arm
tended to do wonky things during some exercises. On
bench press, for example, I was subconsciously
overcompensating for the shoulder, throwing some of the
weight of the lift into my triceps instead, and as a result, I
had stronger triceps on the left side rather than on the
right, my dominant side. My left shoulder was also
noticeably weaker than my right, more so than any other
muscle group on that side of my body.

The surgery was a success; I have no trace of arthritis left
in that shoulder. But my left shoulder is still noticeably
weaker than my right, and I will never, because of this, be
able to bench press David as I had hoped.

## 25

I waited six months to write this. It's about periods. Not the punctuation mark, either.

When I wrote this in 2011, I had suffered from some form of exercise-related amenorrhea since June 2009.

Notice this was not a "confession." This was not an awful truth I'd been hiding. Instead, I was waiting until I felt educated and had this resolved enough to be able to say something intelligent and thoughtful.

Before you jump to conclusions, here's the back story:

I started weight lifting sometime around the beginning of June 2009. About halfway through that month, I did get a normal period. And then I didn't get one in July. Or August. And normally, I was a pretty regular, 30-35 day cycle girl. I couldn't understand why I suddenly had problems—I was not losing weight (I was around 127 when I started weightlifting and was about 122 after 4-5 months of training), and I was not cutting calories.

In August of 2009, I saw the PA in my OB's office (I always see the PA. She's really good, she's a midwife, and she comes highly recommended). I thought she was going to lambaste both my training and my diet. She did neither of those things. Instead, she put me on a birth control pill to regulate my hormones. After some trial and error, I found one form of birth control that seemed to work for me with minimal side effects—the ring.

The ring turned out to be wonderful. I loved it. I had regular periods, though they hardly existed (try three days! woot!), and I didn't have to worry about what appeared to be exercise-related amenorrhea.

Around June of 2010, I started experiencing increasingly bad stomach issues—bloating mostly, though accompanied by other gastrointestinal complaints. I spent all of that summer experimenting with food to figure it out—more fiber? More carbs? Fewer carbs? Less wheat? None of it helped for more than a week.

Finally, in November 2010, I decided to try going off the birth control to see if it was related to my stomach problems. I stopped the ring during the week of Thanksgiving, had a withdrawal period, and waited.

And I waited. And I waited. And I waited.

While I was waiting for my period to come back on its own, I put on about 12 pounds during my massing phase. I was eating more food, more carbs, and more fat, and I was doing far less cardio. My stomach issues improved somewhat, though they never fully went away, but my period never came back.

By the end of May 2011, six months later, I could tell my hormones were stirring around. My skin broke out like I was 15 years old, and it didn't get better in a hurry. I still, however, had no period, so I visited my OB's office again.

This time, I specifically asked the PA about exercise-related amenorrhea. I had often read—not always from highly reputable sources, I will admit—that using birth control as a means of regulating one's hormones in these kinds of cases was just a patch, a quick fix, and not a true cure for the problem. From what I'd read, the only "cure" for amenorrhea was modifying diet or training volume or both—eat more carbs, eat more dietary fat, train less.

None of these options made a lot of sense, I thought, in my case. I didn't develop amenorrhea because of over-training or calorie-reduction. I picked up a barbell, and six weeks later, despite being at the same weight and eating the same number of calories, I had lost my period.

The PA actually agreed with me. She suggested two possible courses of action—start a dose of progesterone to induce a period, wait and see if the hormones regulated themselves, and if not, just keep doing a dose of progesterone every 90ish days. To compensate for the missing estrogen, I could use topical estrogen cream in the meantime.

That all sounded very menopausal to me, and I didn't want to spend every 90 days wondering if I'd get a period and when. So I went with option number two—go back to the ring. This time, the PA prescribed a clinical grade probiotic to help counter some of the possible stomach issues I used to have. With the ring, I would know when I was getting a period every month, there'd be no waiting around for a period to "kick in," and there'd be no need to use estrogen cream since there was a small dose of estrogen in the ring itself. Three weeks after starting the ring again, as well as the probiotic, everything was perfect. No stomach problems, no worrying about if the hormones will regulate themselves.

I was still wondering why it was OK to use birth control to regulate this, though, especially after I'd read so much indicating that this was not the way to handle it. The PA said she wasn't sure where I'd read that, but in her estimation and according to her research, if the birth control would regulate my periods, and therefore reduce my risk of cancer, and the estrogen in it would benefit my bones, and therefore help prevent osteoporosis, there was no reason or evidence that birth control was not a solution to the problem.

I have since tried to assess what her additional reasoning may have been, and so far, this is what I could come up with:

- I was not underweight when the problem started. Nor was I over-training.
- I did gain weight while the problem persisted. No period resulted.
- I was not over-training.

- My diet was not extraordinarily low in any macronutrient, nor was it extremely low in calories (though "low" in calories is relative and dependent on the person in question).
- I did not appear to have what's called the "female athlete triad," or amenorrhea accompanied by low bone density and an eating disorder. In fact, the absence of menses was my *only* symptom.

I finally decided to write about this because I thought it pertinent to our well-being as women who train hard. I suspect many women have been taught the same things I was. I was convinced I was going to be forced to scale back, despite feeling like I wasn't overdoing anything, which I kind of resented. Is amenorrhea, in a woman who is not working for competitive leanness or not suffering an eating disorder, always a sign of overtraining? Or is this a blanket rule applied to women universally, a rule that, in all reality, needs to be evaluated instead on an individual basis?

I worry not all doctors would be as thoughtful as it seems mine was—would other doctors simply tell patients to cut back, even if there was no evidence of over-training other than the lack of menses? Would other doctors simply apply the universal rule in all cases? Has this ever been an issue for anyone else? How was it resolved? Did doctors recommend changes to training and diet, or was birth control used as an option?

Anything I say here applies to me and only me. What is right for me will not be right for someone else, especially if that someone else has medical complications and severe symptoms that I do not. If you have experienced this, please see a doctor. Your treatment will not be the same as mine, nor should it, and I hope you get the same individualized treatment plan that my doctor provided me.

## *26*

How do you know when something is causing you anxiety? Are you always aware of it?

I'm not. Sometimes my brain fools me into thinking there's nothing to worry about, there's no subconscious crisis, and it takes a series of oddly coincidental but somehow related events to show me the light.

For me, it was once a dream that did it. Yes, a dream.

Let me make it clear—I don't usually remember my dreams. I used to swear I didn't dream at all because I never could recall anything other than the occasional nightmare. But a few years ago, on a Thursday night, I had a really clear dream, one with obvious personal implications.

I was, in my dream, a teacher at my old high school. Apparently, I had been teaching there for a while, because I was coming into school for the first time to start the new school year as if I'd been teaching in that building for years. I walked into the building with a colleague, discussing our summers and our new school year as if this was an annual ritual. And I got to the second floor and turned on to a hallway toward a classroom as if I knew exactly what classroom I was going to enter.

When I got to that classroom and took out my key to unlock the door, I realized, as I looked through the door's window, it was my old Math classroom—the room of my favorite high school teacher, Mr. Soffin, the man who originally inspired me to choose teaching, the man who signed my yearbook at the end of senior year and wrote that I was like a daughter to him, the man who was so influential to me that I spent 2 years tutoring his Algebra students during my study halls after I'd already moved into Pre-Calc and AP Calc with another Math teacher.

As I looked into the classroom from the outside, I saw that everything in his room was exactly as I remembered it—the teacher desk was where it always was, the desks were overcrowding the space, and the rows were exactly as he'd have them. It was still his space, not mine, and I immediately felt I wasn't worthy of using it. I couldn't, in my dream, even unlock the door—instead, I stood outside his room and bawled my eyes out, mourning that fact that I wasn't the teacher that he had been, that I hadn't lived up to my ideal.

That's when I woke up.

Obviously, my shift away from teaching high school full-time to pursuing a nutrition-related degree was causing me some subconscious anxiety that summer. Somewhere, in the back of my head, the possibility that this pursuit of fitness & nutrition might cause me to leave teaching behind was akin to saying I was an unsuccessful teacher, akin to saying, by pursuing something else, that I wasn't a good teacher. In my dream, I wasn't worthy of inhabiting the same space as Mr. Soffin, and I was, therefore, a disappointment to both myself and everything he represented.

I woke up that Friday morning and felt kind of sad. I had been having a great time, all week, pursuing my non-teaching interests. I'd had great workouts all week, I was finally genuinely enjoying my Chemistry labs, and I managed to get my best grade of the course on my last Chemistry unit quiz that week. It all made me look forward with excitement to the Nutrition classes I'd be starting at the end of the month. But the dream seemed to crush it all—what good was my enjoyment of all those things if I wasn't living up to being the person, the teacher, I'd always thought I wanted to be?

I spent Friday feeling kind of numb. I wasn't really sure how to make myself feel better, other than to wait. And think a lot.

The next morning, as always, my alarms (I have 3!) went off, and I rolled over to hit snooze on all of them. Even my phone was set with a daily alarm, and I hit snooze on that as well. I happened to have a few emails and Facebook notifications too, so in my half-asleep daze, I read through what was on my phone. One message, in particular, sent late Friday night from a reader of my blog, woke me up in a hurry:

*I really need to say thank you to you. You have no idea what your blog did for me. I read your period post, and it got me thinking. I have not had a regular period for a few years and have always contributed it [sic] to my exercise. However, this summer I have been getting bad acne right around my period time—which is very strange for me. After reading your blog, I decided to see what my options were with the doctor. The last thing I wanted to do was go on birth control, but I also wanted my hormones to be under control. So last Tuesday, I went to my regular doctor who sent me to an OB/GYN. I went there on Thursday, had blood work done on Friday, then two days ago (Wednesday), I had a sonogram which showed that I had a massive cyst—14cm. After more blood work yesterday, it showed that I really needed to get that sucker out. So this morning I went in and had it removed. While they were in there, they found another 14cm cyst right next to it. Unfortunately, through all this, I lost one of my ovaries. However, if this had not been caught sooner, there could have been a lot worse results. I am sorry for giving you my medical history, but as I am trying to get comfortable with the stitches, I was reminded how I probably never would have gone to the doctor if I had not read your post. So thank you, for real.*

I almost cried.

For real this time, not in a dream, and not because I was mourning what I thought was a lack of achievement on my part.

This time, I almost cried out of genuine satisfaction—something I had done, something I had decided to write, had helped someone in a truly significant way.

Even more significantly, the blog post this message refers to was a difficult one for me to write—I was afraid, when I wrote that post about my own problems with amenorrhea, that I would be lambasted with comments advising me to "get healthy" or insisting I absolutely MUST change my diet or training. Just as I was reluctant to post all of the details of my food plans because of the critiques I'd seen other bloggers deal with, I was reluctant to discuss my problems with amenorrhea for similar reasons.

In the end, however, discussing the issues surrounding exercise-related amenorrhea was far more important than possibly taking some critiques in reader comments. I was sure of my body, my diet, and my training, and I was confident in the treatment course I'd chosen with my doctor. I knew I could stand by the personal decisions I'd already made and that writing that post was more about bringing up an often undiscussed issue than it was about defending myself.

Once the amenorrhea post was published, the comments I received from readers reassured me right away that I'd made the right decision in posting it. And the heartfelt email from that reader sealed that confidence.

But that reader email happened to come at the exact right time—right in my moment of existential crisis—and showed that, even if I was not a classroom teacher, what I do could still have a profound effect on the lives of the people around me.

I still had no idea where my pursuit of fitness and nutrition, or that Nutrition degree, was going to lead; I could, in a few years, still have been a teacher. Or I could not be.

Regardless of what I actually was, though, the dream and the reader message made me see what was really at issue was what I "do"—whose life changed as a result of my guidance or experience. In the end, isn't that what I wanted, at heart, when I became a teacher?

I had always thought my goal in life was to be the "teacher" Mr. Soffin had been in the classroom.

Today my goal is to be the "teacher" he was in life.

And I can do that under whatever title, teacher or otherwise, I choose.

## 27

In January 2012, I got a side gig was a personal trainer, and as of March 8th, 2012, I had officially been a trainer for about eight weeks.

That's not a long time, but it was long enough to have a few random observations to help tell the story of my experiences at that point.

*Almost Vomiting*

That'd be me who almost vomited, not my clients. I was more nervous before my first official training session than I was during either of the interviews that got me the job in the first place. Maybe that's because job interviews were old hat to me. I can't tell you the number of teaching interviews I've been on, and if you've ever interviewed for a teaching job, you know what those are like.

My nerves went away as soon as I had my client doing her first exercise, but holy crap. I could have puked. Several times.

*People Need to Talk*

I had a handful of clients who didn't want to be pushed too hard, a handful who worked their asses off, and a handful who were right in between. But they all seemed to have one thing in common: they had a better workout—and seemed to push themselves harder—if they were given a chance to talk.

I don't mean spending the entire session talking instead of working. I watched trainers at another local gym do this, and it drove me nuts because clients aren't paying for a friendly chat.

However, having a few seconds to talk about dinner, or children, or frustrations, or the interesting story on the news seemed to give many people the level of comfort needed to be willing to crank out a strong set.

This only seems logical to me; clients didn't really know me. For all they knew, I might be spending my Sunday afternoons dressed as a Star Trek character. Or taking needlepoint classes. Why would I expect that a client would trust my direction and my estimation of his/her abilities if I hadn't established some sort of personal rapport first?

Clients with whom I had established some social ease progressed faster and worked harder. Good classroom teachers know this is the case with students as well.

*I Was Now Fair Game for Questions*

I stopped wearing headphones at the gym.

First, after working with a trainer for 3 years, I had grown accustomed to lifting with someone nearby, so music had been an afterthought.

Second, even when I lifted alone, my mp3 player's clip had broken off months ago. No more attaching it to my waistband. And I don't like armbands.

I even tried tucking my mp3 player into my sports bra, not caring about the fact that this made me look like I had a small rectangular growth on my left boob. But try deadlifting with that in your shirt. Or try doing squat thrusts like that. It fell out. I didn't have the boobage to keep it in.

Plus, having the mp3 player in my shirt meant that I would often accidentally touch it and hit the repeat button—lying leg curls and lat pulldowns often did this.

So no more headphones for me.

That left me open to questions from gym members while I was working out.

Once, a guy whom I'd often seen in the weight area asked me about the sumo deadlifts I was doing. *What muscle groups do they work? If I do back and legs separately, when could I incorporate them?*

I was more than happy to answer questions. And I'd often see my own clients while I was working out. It gave me good exposure to gym members anyway, so I considered all this a positive and a possible way to get & retain clients.

## Even Beginners Get Frustrated

This was perhaps the most important thing I learned.

I once had a client cry. Not because of something I did or an injury. Instead, she had specific wrist and knee limitations due to rheumatoid arthritis, and we discovered that, on DB shoulder presses, her left arm failed. Fast.

This was a client who always tried her hardest—if she could do it, she did do it, despite it feeling like hard work. So she tried repeatedly to make that left arm do what she wanted.

And after 10 or 12 tries, mostly failures, she broke down.

And I had to fix it.

I told her that we could work around it, that we would get her shoulder workout in via another exercise that would be just as effective. And I told her my own stories of frustrating post-surgery limitations and days when my body just refused to do what my brain told it to do.

So we did what I said—we worked around it. We did something else, and she worked her butt off. But she'd been dealing with the discrepancy between her body and her brain for a while. I knew, despite the fact that our workout turned out OK, she was still beating herself up for it when she left that day.

That day reminded me of how personal this is for people—training is not just something to get done and out of the way for some clients. Just like when I started out myself, for some of my clients, there are very real, tangible goals attached to these workouts. When those goals get postponed or thwarted by things that can't be easily controlled, it sucks.

I get that.

I totally get it.

And I'm a better trainer for having learned it.

## *28*

March 2012 had another milestone for me.

I stopped being a vegetarian.

Pick up your jaws.

Got 'em yet?

I'll wait.

Now let me answer the 1756 questions you might have.

**Question #1. Why?**

A) I was having some stomach issues and was 90% sure they were related to eating an awful lot of dairy, specifically cottage cheese, which lead me to believe I had issues digesting casein. I spent February 2012 researching casein, and sure enough, most of my stomach problems were textbook casein issues—slow digestion, slow motility, and bloating. I wasn't having "allergic" reactions to dairy, as in no rash, eczema, or asthma. And I didn't believe it was lactose intolerance because the symptoms just didn't match. Casein intolerance seemed likely.

B) I could no longer eat soy. Soy, in most forms, gave me instant stomach problems and migraines. As soon as I gave up tofu in 2011, I saw great improvements in the digestive issues I was suffering. They never fully dissipated (perhaps because of the cottage cheese still in my diet), but eating even a small bit of soy—like vegetables roasted in soybean oil—reminded me within an hour of why I gave it up. I, therefore, couldn't replace cottage cheese with soy protein.

C) I was already eating eggs and egg whites 2-3 times a day. I loved eggs and egg whites, but I remembered the day I prepped for my SIBO test before this. I ate eggs six times that day. Who the eff wants to do that all the time?

D) I also spent significant amounts of time researching seafood as a protein source. I looked at mercury-content lists. I'd been to the Wegmans website many times searching for wild-caught, low-fat options. There was even a morning where I went into the store to buy Greek yogurt and found myself on the tuna fish aisle for a good 12-15 minutes. I read every single can and package label on that aisle.

(Did you know, for example, that some of those foil-packed tunas are doused in vegetable broth made from soy? Read the labels carefully if you're avoiding soy.)

*So I did my homework.*

**Question #2. How did this start?**

When I had a small piece of Pacific cod for dinner one night.

It was relatively good—I was a little surprised, to be honest, that it wasn't "fishy" as I seem to recall seafood being when I was a kid. I drizzled some mushroom & sage olive oil over it, seasoned it with Mrs. Dash's Onion & Herb blend, baked it for 20 minutes, and topped it with salsa.

And even though I forgot that fish shrinks when it is cooked and was therefore worried that a mere 4 ounces wouldn't keep me full for long, I wound up feeling more satiated than I would have had I eaten egg whites instead.

*Go figure.*

After that, I tried tuna at lunch and cod once again for dinner.

## Question #3. Did you eat other animals? Like mammals?

I wasn't sure, at first, if I would.

My goal was to simply cut cottage cheese back as much as possible and to limit Greek yogurt and whey to one serving each per day if possible. Once I saw how that went, I would reassess.

I did eventually add meat back in, and today I eat mostly beef, chicken, and turkey for all of my meals.

**Question #4. Did you get sick from the fish?**

Nope!

It is a myth that we lose the ability to digest animal protein when we become vegetarian or vegan. Besides, I had been eating animal protein in the form of eggs and dairy all along. Some people who make the transition might feel a little stomach discomfort at first, especially if, like me, they have been vegan or vegetarian for more than a little while.

Until that day in 2012, it had been 14 years since I'd eaten seafood. Maybe longer since it wasn't part of my regular diet even when I did eat meat. But after dinner that night, I had a little stomach tightness—for lack of a better word—and within about an hour, I felt fine.

And the day after, I felt even better.

It wasn't just because of one seafood meal that I felt great. Cutting cottage cheese caused much of my bloating to go away. My stomach felt good—not full, heavy, or thick-feeling all the time. My obliques even came back after a short hiatus. And this is not a question of having lost fat, either; my calorie and macro intake were the same. It's just that my protein sources were changing.

## Question #5. Were you worried what people would think?

The only person whose opinion I considered in this process was David's. I was kind of worried he wouldn't like me anymore if I wasn't still vegetarian—our shared vegetarianism was something we had always valued, and David has never eaten meat or seafood in his life.

We talked that weekend, however, and he was more than supportive. This was not a decision he would've made, but he recognized that

> a) I was never a vegetarian for ethical reasons in the first place, and

> b) we already used animal products, and I could make this food transition in responsible ways.

I can't tell you how relieved I was to know he was OK with this.

But aside from David, no one else's opinion was relevant in this decision. This was a question of my health, my quality of life, and my individual volition. Nothing else.

And those things—health, quality of life, and individual volition—are the best reasons I can think of to make this kind of change.

## *29*

There was one blog post I wasn't sure I would ever publish.

I needed, however, to write it. I needed BADLY to write it. I needed to flesh out, on paper, or in digital space, at least, exactly what had been happening in my head, stomach, body, and heart for the first four months of 2012.

It started during the week between Christmas Eve and New Year's Eve 2011. During the week before those holidays, I weighed a little over 116 pounds. I was feeling super good—I was sleeping 7-8 hours a night, sticking to my macros, not drinking alcohol, working out 6-7 days a week, and recovering well. I had just finished my PT cert and was job hunting. And Christmas was my favorite holiday.

As usual, I ate whatever I wanted on Christmas Eve. Pizza and cookies, mostly. And then more cookies. And more cookies. And a few more cookies before bed.

I ate conservatively all morning on Christmas, then again ate whatever I wanted as I visited various family members throughout the day. And once again, I topped it off with more cookies before bed.

All of that sounds like a lot, but really, I hadn't eaten like that in forever. And I was in great shape otherwise, so my two-day holiday food festivities wouldn't make a huge dent in whatever I was trying to accomplish.

Even the pizza and cake and cookies and whiskey I had on New Year's Eve wasn't a big deal in the grand scheme of things.

But come post-holiday time, it was hard to stay on track. I found myself overeating a little bit every day—most days it was just some extra cottage cheese, extra greek yogurt, maybe a few extra tablespoons of peanut butter.

Sometimes, on a Sunday night (for some reason these nights were a weak spot for me), it'd be more than just a "little" extra dairy and peanut butter. It was half jars of peanut butter. Full containers of cottage cheese. Several handfuls of raw nuts if we had them in the house.

At some point in February or March, my food of choice turned into bread, not just dairy or nuts. The first time I binged on bread I was disgusted with myself afterward— was it six slices I'd had? Seven? Did I count the whole wheat banana muffin I'd eaten in between rounds of bread? And what about the coconut oil I was putting on it?

In whole, I couldn't really recount the number of times I binged on food during those months. If I were to guess, I'd estimate that it was 2-3 times a week, sometimes more than once on a binge day. Vulnerable times of day seemed to be late afternoon (3-4 PM) and late evening (9-10 PM) for me.

That didn't mean that I was only overeating during those hours; there was a Friday morning at school—of all places—where I sat at my desk unwrapping snack-sized chocolate bars, eating them during my prep period and while my students did their silent reading.

And I am pretty sure I went home and binged on more bread that afternoon.

By April of 2012, I weighed somewhere in the neighborhood of 131 pounds. That was fifteen pounds since Christmas.

I originally thought that I just had problems with specific foods—that I needed to stop eating peanut butter, for example. But it seemed like that was only replacing one "bad" food with another—and what I needed was simply control, not a long list of foods to avoid.

So how did I get that?

How did I regain control over something I thought I was already in control of? And how did I avoid returning to binge eating in the future?

I decided there were several things I should do.

1. I had to admit this was my choice.

I was not going to pretend stress, lack of sleep, too much work, or some deep-rooted insecurities weren't part of the reason behind my binges.

But regardless of those influences, and despite the paralysis that accompanies a binge, I chose what food I did or did not eat. I chose bread. I chose a lot of it. I chose chocolate. I chose peanut butter in obscene quantities.

I could also, therefore, choose NOT to make those same decisions again.

2. I bought new gym clothes that do not fit and kept them.

I didn't do this on purpose. I have this habit of buying new gym clothes without trying them on. Then I get home to see if I like them, and usually, they're fine. I return the few exceptions whenever I get a chance, but 90% of my purchases fit just great.

Until I gained 15 pounds. I bought a few shirts and two pairs of shorts that were just a little too snug for comfort. And one shirt that outright made me look like I'd stuffed myself into a kid's size.

I rarely used this kind of motivation for myself, but I kept those gym clothes rather than returning them. Because had I not chosen to eat this way, these clothes would have fit with no problem.

3. I gave up wheat.

Binge eating in any way made me feel sick, literally, but binge eating wheat products made me feel incredibly sick. The symptoms of post-wheat-binge-sickness were rather interesting and disturbing all at once:

- Nausea when I finally started to feel hungry again.
- Nasty bloat that didn't start until about an hour post-binge.
- Horrible gas a few hours post-bloat, sometimes lasting into the next day, meaning the wheat wasn't digesting properly in my system.
- Several post-bloat bathroom trips that were less than happy or pretty.

Sorry for the graphics, but this was the post that was never going to get published, right?

I'll say it bluntly then:

High quantities of wheat turned my intestines into shit. Literally.

4. I admitted that I was prone to addictions.

I guess I should've known that about myself when I smoked a pack of cigarettes a day for 10 years, huh?

If I could quit smoking, I could stop binge eating.

5. I slowly dieted my way back to normal.

Slowly meant no crash diet, no severe restrictions. I ate carbs. I ate lots of protein, and I had fun trying new proteins in the process.

I cooked my first grass-fed steak in my post-binge-eating period.

I planned on trying pork chops. And I hoped to love them.

One might think, by the way, that a "diet" is a poor way to stop a binge eater, especially a binge eater who was doing all this while she was supposed to be following her macros.

But I have done plenty of thinking about why I started the binges to begin with, and I don't think it was from diet frustration. It certainly wasn't a rebound from extreme restriction, either. So I knew a moderate plan and some accountability will be helpful.

6. I did not saddle myself with guilt.

I didn't see how guilt would be productive. Why would it be good to make myself feel awful and remorseful for having eaten food? Wouldn't that just eff up whatever relationship I had with food even more? Make me associate eating with guilt?

Eating is healthy.

Guilt would compromise that.

I could admit my choices were poor ones without bombarding myself with feelings of self-resentment.

I may have been an asshole for doing this to myself, but I refused to be defined as an asshole by holding a ridiculous grudge against myself.

7. I set performance-based gym goals to avoid focus on losing body fat.

Was I trying to lose the body fat I just accumulated?

Fuck yes.

But I did not make it the goal of my workouts.

It seemed healthy to separate diet from the gym then. Let the food and macros do their work. Keep the workout focus on achievement instead.

I set my sights on chin-ups, not fat loss.

8. I had to acknowledge all this publicly.

I was not sure anyone fully knew about this. Not even David. Binge eating is not something you do with witnesses—I often waited for David to go out, or to take a nap, and did my binging then. And binge eating certainly isn't something you readily tell people about, even friends.

So if you're my friend, or my boot camp buddy, or my parent, or my brother, or my coach, or my former student, or my workout partner, or my internet-friend, my apologies for not being upfront about this.

It is hard to admit when you're struggling—I have always had issues with asking for help.

And binge eating is an awfully lonely act.

9. I recognized that even those of us with a dedication to fitness, those of us who pride ourselves on being extraordinarily self-motivated, could still suffer from disordered eating, even for short periods.

I can't fathom the idea that even professional fitness competitors aren't troubled by bouts with disordered eating. They must be.

And if they aren't, well, good for them. But lots of other fitness professionals ARE plagued by this.

Count me among them.

But then count me among those who got past it.

## *30*

Sunday was normally a problematic night for me. I'd have some time to myself to do nothing, and for four months in 2012, this was often a time when I found myself in the midst of a binge before I knew what was happening.

Sunday nights were some kind of auto-binge-trigger for me. Maybe it was the disappointment that the weekend was over—only teachers *truly* know the pain of a Sunday evening. Maybe it was the lack of a long to-do list—on weeknights, I'd get home from either work or boot camp between 8 and 9 PM and still have to eat something, prep breakfast, relax for 20 seconds, and get my ass into bed.

Sunday nights felt different. They felt quiet. They felt long. And they felt empty.

In an attempt to be proactive, I set out to establish a new Sunday normal. It'd been a while since I spent the afternoon food prepping for the week, so I went back to that habit.

I spent entire afternoons roasting sweet potatoes, butternut squash, acorn squash, cauliflower, Brussels sprouts, and fennel. I made David a Greek pasta salad to use for lunch for the week, and I made myself a few above average meals to keep myself happy. I usually resorted to eggs and canned tuna on Sunday afternoons, mostly out of ease and general laziness, but I switched my proteins for new options to keep myself interested.

With all that food prep done, and all those veggies waiting around to be eaten, the idea of binge eating ANYTHING seemed wrong. I didn't know if Sunday food prep would always keep me from a binge, but when I first tried to stop binge eating, it helped.

In general, though, just keeping my brain and body busy was a good thing. So I made myself a long list of things with which to occupy myself:

*Warning: none of these is interesting in the least.*

Read. Watch *Food Network*. Call my mom. (Hi, Mom.) Fold laundry.

Boring, I know. Incredibly mundane.

But that's what I needed on my new Sunday nights.

## *31*

Are you familiar with behavior theory?

How about the transtheoretical model of behavior change?

Here are the basics:

Behavior change happens in stages—you start with pre-contemplation, in which you don't want to or even consider change, then you contemplate change, then you prepare for change, then you put change into action, then you either maintain change or regress and have to restart the cycle all over again.

Although if you regress and start again, this cycle might start to feel more like banging your head against a wall.

This is exactly how I felt one week in May of 2012. Like I had been willingly banging my own forehead against a wall.

Repeatedly.

I had a binge relapse the week before, right after I wrote about how great I was doing with controlling my bread intake. Despite my best efforts to not beat myself up over the binge, I did beat myself up.

A lot.

This took the form, mostly, of self-analysis, repeatedly thinking about what I had eaten, extra time spent awake in bed when I should've been sleeping, and a few days of being extra bitchy.

Notice what it didn't entail—no binges as a result of the binge.

That is a good thing, but the relapse, while perhaps normal, wasn't a good thing.

What did I eat?

Bread, and David's jar of peanut butter.

UGH.

Because of this, I ran out of Ezekiel bread. And then I went grocery shopping that weekend and stood in the bread and peanut butter aisle (yeah, they're in the same aisle in my store), wondering if I should buy either item again.

I didn't.

Well, sort of. We bought peanut butter for David but no second jar for me. And no bread for me.

I wondered if this was how it worked. You resolve just to eat your problem food in moderation, find you can't, resolve not to eat it at all, find that you can't, resolve to eat it in moderation, find that you can't, resolve not to eat it at all…

Endless vicious cycle?

I didn't want that to happen. I hadn't the patience for that. I didn't relapse when I quit smoking, not once. So this was new to me. I didn't know what to do with it.

Except to move on. Stop the brick-wall-head-banging. Stop the over-analysis.

Stop even thinking about the relapse at all.

Done.

## *32*

I felt like a recovering addict.

Later on, I finally felt "normal."

"Normal" meant a lot of things, in this case.

For example, my brain didn't feel super foggy.

I didn't know whether it was the last binge, the content of that binge (lots of things, but lots of bread), or the emotional low that resulted from it. Regardless, my head hadn't been in the game since then, despite my efforts that night to put binges behind me.

After my weekend of debating whether to buy bread and peanut butter, the following Tuesday was terribly difficult for me. I had set my binge eating confession post to publish while I was off at boot camp. It was scheduled to go live at 7 PM.

At one point, I happened to turn around and check the clock at boot camp to see how much time we had left. It was 7:05. My heart skipped a little beat. The post was out there, and I could do nothing about it.

After boot camp, I really just wanted to go to bed. But I had some things to deal with that couldn't wait. I had to tell my trainer about the binges before he read it on my blog. I had to eat some dinner before bed, too, and I had to avoid letting that dinner turn into yet another binge.

And, in what turned out to be the best part of that night, I had a lot of positive reader comments and Facebook messages to respond to after that post. I couldn't have asked for a more supportive response from any of you that night.

Even the day after, though, my brain was still in a cloud. I went to bed extra early just to let myself rest, and I was sound asleep by 9:45 the next night.

I felt better and clearer after a few days.

If you've ever read Sylvia Plath's *The Bell Jar*, you know the main character, Esther, undergoes electroshock therapy several times, and finally, when the procedure is done correctly, she feels some relief from the suffocating "bell jar," her depression, that's been hanging over her. She says, "The bell jar hung, suspended, a few feet above my head. I was open to the circulating air."

I'm no mental patient as Esther was, but as cliché as it sounds, I felt as though a weight had been lifted. I felt a little less burdened. And that was a good start.

My body is also felt a little lighter, a little happier. My hunger signals returned between meals. I'm not sure if this happens when others binge, but I would lose clear hunger signals for a few days post-binge. My body knows it's stuffed, so my brain doesn't trigger eating cues as it normally would.

Even now, as I was just typing that part about Esther from *The Bell Jar*, I felt a familiar empty rumble in my stomach. And it made me happy.

We seem to spend so much of our lives avoiding feeling a little hungry—we think it's a bad thing to feel hunger pangs, stomach rumbles, or the slightest angst of not yet having eaten. But hunger signals can be healthy things. They're hormonal cues from your brain not only saying it's time to eat, but your internal system of checks and balances is working.

They also help you distinguish between hunger (a physical state) and appetite (a psychological state).

Can you experience hunger signals even when your body's system of checks and balances is unhealthy or out of whack? Sure. But I welcomed those hunger signals. And I was happy to be eating to fulfill hunger, not appetite.

Despite the positives, I was sure the next few weeks, maybe even months, were going to be a struggle in some ways. I was sure that I would face more difficult days than I had already experienced.

But I went forward with every bit of self-awareness that I could.

That made me hopeful. And it made that day, finally, a good day.

## *33*

I remember April 24, 2012, very well.

It was a Tuesday, and I was at school teaching. I'd spent four months wrestling with uncharacteristic binge eating habits, and I was fed up with myself and with food. I spent much of my free period writing a post about it, "coming clean" to my readers, that I didn't think I'd publish. Then I emailed it to a fellow blogger, whose response helped me decide:

I needed to publish it. I needed to be honest. So I set my post to publish at around 7 PM when I would be in a boot camp class and likely in the midst of doing 732 squat thrusts.

By the time I left boot camp, there were already responses to the post—and they were encouraging, supportive, thankful, and just as honest as my post had been. The responses convinced me I'd done the right thing by writing that post. And they also showed me that even the most "fit" women—and men—struggle with overeating and binge eating behaviors.

Even now, I can't help but think of that night. I remember boot camp that evening because I was nervous, anxious, and concerned. I had put my entire reputation as a fitness and nutrition blogger on the line to openly express the very real problems I was experiencing with something that had always been easy for me—controlling my eating habits.

What if my readers thought I was a fake? What if I couldn't get this problem under control? Would I have to stop blogging? Change my blog's name from *Following Fit* to *Following Food*?

I left boot camp that night feeling empty, but not in a good, purged, restarting kind of way. I had gotten my problems off my chest, but I still felt like something, some part of me, was missing.

Writing that post might have been the right thing to do, but it didn't change whatever the problem was that was causing my behaviors.

I spent a lot of the next year working on my behaviors with regard to food—I wrote about it, and wrote about it, and wrote about it, but I never really seemed to get anywhere, even after reading books like *Breaking the Binge*, until I was honest with myself about why I was behaving this way.

I had always had a strong sense of personal identity, even in the face of most change, before my eating problems. I was a teacher, a blogger, a weightlifter. I was motivated, I had no demons, and I never thought twice about food other than following my macros.

When I started the switch away from teaching and into the fitness field, however, I lost something. I lost part of who I thought I was—a teacher—and was attempting to replace it with something I wasn't sure I was—a trainer.

In short, I didn't know myself anymore.

It's probably not a coincidence these binges began around Christmas of 2011, just as I was trying to find a job as a trainer. It's probably not a coincidence this came to an emotional head when I realized, sometime around April of 2012, that I needed to take a break from teaching.

I was just lost. And I don't mean just that I was unsure of my career.

I mean some significant part, maybe several parts, of who I believed myself to be was missing. A big old hunk of Kristen had disappeared.

All of my attempts to relearn new food habits, to write about my habits, to break the cycle—all of those things couldn't truly keep me from binge eating. Any time I felt like I didn't know who I was, my habits returned.

I used to think of the binge eating problem as compensation for stress. I always knew I wasn't doing it out of the typical dissatisfaction with a restrictive diet. I didn't realize, however, that it wasn't truly about simple stress.

It was about identity.

I used to be the girl who never ate emotionally, but when I lost my sense of self, I became an emotional eater. It was as if, because one part of my self was gone, it was all gone—including my control over food.

It wasn't until 2013, a year after admitting my issues, however, that I started to think of it this way. It finally occurred to me one day, when I was feeling the urge to eat, that something more than stress, something more than simply eating out of habit, was going on. In fact, what seemed to trigger the urge to eat that day was another identity crisis, namely a sense of regret over not being the person I used to be—the person who *didn't* binge.

Having realized this, 2013 felt like the end of a long, long road for me.

I could have felt like shit about myself—I hadn't lost the weight I gained over that last year, I was slower and had to work harder in boot camp than I used to, and I knew I hadn't treated myself well, neither while in the throes of a binge nor while attempting to forgive myself for what had already happened.

But instead of feeling awful, I felt really good. I felt strong. I felt like I had finished something huge, the first step in a positive process. And I felt something even better, something I hadn't felt in a long time, and something I wasn't sure I would feel again:

I felt whole.

## *34*

I also distinctly remember Easter Day 2012.

Well, sort of.

I *think* I worked at the gym in the morning; I had a few Sunday morning clients since I started there that January. And I *think* I did hamstrings afterward since up until a few months before that, that was my lifting schedule for about a year.

Despite these uncertainties, I *do* distinctly remember these two things:

*Feeling and looking absolutely exhausted from my work schedule.*

I was seriously beaten up—physically and emotionally—by Easter that year. I had been teaching part-time, personal training part-time, going to grad school full-time, and pulling my hair out trying to stop myself from binge eating once or twice a week. I think my mother might have even told me I looked awful on Easter. Or tired. Or something like that.

Regardless, it was true—I did look tired and exhausted.

I had the week following Easter off from teaching and needed it badly—but I also remember going back to teaching after the break and not feeling one bit more refreshed than when I left.

By the following Easter, I wasn't so stressed. No binge eating. No overeating. And I looked like I'd slept more than three hours a night that week.

*Eating whatever the eff I wanted that day because I thought it didn't matter.*

I don't know when or if I binged in the week preceding Easter 2012, but I do remember feeling like watching what I ate on Easter was a waste of time and energy.

So I had ham (even though I didn't love it). I had scalloped potatoes (which I will always love). I had seconds. And I am pretty sure I had chocolate of some kind at some point.

I also remember this:

I didn't enjoy any of it. I just felt it was useless NOT to eat it.

I felt trapped by the new binge habits I was developing. It felt utterly futile to resist those habits, despite how much I wanted to change them. So my answer, that day, was to feed that misery with more food, food I didn't even love.

It's no coincidence I finally posted something about my binge eating just three weeks after Easter of 2012, and it's no coincidence I remember that Easter so well. That Easter was one of many low points for me—and I had quite a few of those, some of which I remember as clearly as I remember that Easter. It wasn't just the food that made it a low point; it was my entire view of my world at the time.

I don't think I felt I had a single thing to be happy about on that day.

And thinking about that today makes me sad for my previous self.

But it also makes me happy for my current self, who has hundreds of things to be happy about.

## 35

Four months.

That's how long I was binge eating before I confessed I was doing so.

And how long did it take me to really stop binge eating?

*Over three years.*

You see, even though I could say that I was past most of the issues that caused and continued my binge eating issues in 2012, 2013, and early 2014, I don't think that binge eating, or any other disordered eating pattern, is something from which you ever fully recover.

I will always, always have to be cognizant of my former habits.

Recovering from this kind of problem isn't like recovering from the flu. You don't just get to lie around on the couch for 3-5 days, sleep a lot, eat some soup, blow your nose, and then move on. There's no Tamiflu or Z-Pack for binge eating. There's no magic diet to follow, no magic formula about foods to avoid, no miracle workout program.

What worked for me isn't going to work for anyone but me. Recovery, just like the development of binge eating to start with, is personal.

I can't isolate one single thing I think helped me the most. Eating habits are so much a part of the fabric of our lives I can't separate any of the following factors from the rest. They worked as a whole for me, not as steps in a process, and it has only been through the integration of ALL of these things that I have been able to achieve permanent change.

*Practice*

I hate the cliché, here, but it is true:

I had to practice NOT binge eating, all the time, to be able to do so more effortlessly. That sounds reasonable, but there's a problem inherent in "practice" that I had to get past somehow—failure is inevitable.

I failed at practicing a lot, and those failures added up to more weight gains. When I first admitted to the problem in 2012, I had gained 15-20 pounds, and I weighed somewhere around 130-135 pounds. I got all the way up to 155 at one point, and that was well after admitting there was a problem.

That doesn't mean that I was binge eating with the same frequency as when I first began trying to fix the issue. At first, I was binge eating 2-3 days a week, more than once per day on those days. But I began binge eating when I was quite lean and already muscular—meaning I had the metabolic capacity to handle more food easily at first. At some point, though, my body lost some of that insulin sensitivity, precisely because I was still binge eating, and I continued to gain weight even though I was binge eating less.

So every time I failed at practicing more normal eating habits, I was not only reinforcing my brain's proclivity for binge eating, but I was also reinforcing my body's inability to cope with those extra calories—another way in which binge eating can become a vicious cycle.

I persisted in my practice, however, and kept trying to not binge.

*Self-Detachment*

I learned this from reading *Brain Over Binge*.

It wasn't enough to just practice not binge eating. I had to think about my thoughts every time I went to eat food and particularly if I felt I was about to embark on a binge. This kind of meta-analysis does not come naturally. We tend to feel hunger, think food, then eat food, and we never fully stop and question where the initial impetus to eat started.

Every time I thought I wanted to eat, I had to stop and rationalize that urge. Where was it coming from? Was I hungry, for real? Or bored? Or stressed? Or was it triggered by the fact that it was 8 PM on a Sunday night, and my brain was simply habituated to starting a binge right around that time?

That last part—that the brain will trigger a binge as a result of building that behavioral pattern over time—is the part I learned from *Brain Over Binge*. It feels like we cannot resist the binge because the impetus to start eating comes from a deep-rooted, irrational part of the brain, the same part that stores all our other habitual behaviors, healthy and unhealthy.

Rather than follow the impulse, I had to think of that impulse as an outside stimulus—like someone ELSE was suggesting it to me. I had to detach it from its source (within me) and see it as something I could remove from myself.

Once I could detach like that, saying no was like saying no to anything I didn't want, like saying no to a glass of water if I wasn't thirsty.

*Diet Changes*

I didn't want to admit I needed to fix my metabolism.

I was used to being able to eat a lot of food, and I was used to being able to handle refeeds that had lots of carbs. I couldn't even start losing body fat, though, until I admitted that I was going to have to improve my body's ability to handle food first. Admitting that, in combination with improved practice at normal eating, allowed me to start losing some weight in 2014.

At first, I was losing weight with a pretty low-carb diet. No starches, carbs around workouts only, and protein, veggies, and fat the rest of the day. I have since been able to add plenty of carbs back in, and I am continuing to lose body fat, though I would love to see my carb intake improve even more.

That's not to say that everyone will have to go low-carb, and that's not to say that low-carb was the only diet change I had to face.

I also had to wrestle with my trigger foods—bread and peanut butter and baked goods—and I went through several phases of inclusion and exclusion with these foods. I finally concluded that if a food was still triggering a binge, I shouldn't eat it. At all.

I don't see that as deprivation, for anyone who wants to argue that all foods are healthy in moderation.

"Moderation" is an idea that only applies to folks with no food-specific disordered habits.

For those of us with disordered habits tied to specific food items, avoidance is a useful strategy until a new habit can replace the disordered one.

I still didn't eat bread, mostly because of an ongoing issue with eating FODMAPs (and wheat is one), but I delved into peanut butter sometimes.

And I still overate peanut butter from time to time.

But I didn't keep it in my daily meals, and it wasn't easily accessible to me most of the time, and that was purposeful. I wasn't ready to trust myself with peanut butter moderation, but that didn't mean I was somehow less "recovered" from binge eating.

It just means I didn't eat much peanut butter.

*Underlying Causes*

Binge eating is tied to emotional distress of some kind.

At least, it was for me.

I was undergoing a massive identity crisis when I began binge eating. Was I a teacher? A trainer? A writer? A nutritionist?

My ability to do the things I mentioned above—practice, self-detachment, and diet changes—didn't develop until I tackled my identity issues. Ironically, the very thing that triggered my initial issues, which was an absence from teaching, was the trigger that helped solve my issues in 2014.

I went back to teaching.

I made that decision in April 2014, and I still weighed 150+ at the time.

Most of the success I have had in getting back down to the low 130s has happened since I made that career decision. Having a solid sense of who I was contributed to my ability to feel like I could successfully lose body fat—and that most certainly applies to anyone trying to change her body.

How can you have the confidence that you will succeed in something as daunting as body recomposition if you don't have any confidence in who you are overall?

Success is always a choice, and those who have experienced the high of success in some areas are more likely to choose success in others. Just another way in which success—like binge eating—is a cycle.

The more you do it, the more you will continue to do it.

I may never be able to say I am done recovering from binge eating.

But I can say that I am actively feeding my future recovery, building my own success cycle one day at a time.

The more I succeed now, the more I will succeed later.

And that's not a bad deal.

## *36*

Lost yourself? Stop looking, and you'll find yourself.

Let's consult Google to help us define "self" before we get started:

*a person's essential being that distinguishes them from others, especially considered as the object of introspection or reflexive action*

First, let's ignore the erroneous pronoun-antecedent agreement in the definition.

Instead, let's rephrase: the self is that part of you that makes you essentially different from Joe Schmoe on the treadmill next to you.

You can also think of it, as I do, as any number of things:

- self is confidence
- self is mojo
- self is the ability to overcome
- self is essence
- self is drive
- self is a habit
- self is coping
- self is creating

In other words, maybe we can define self as that essential thing—that one essential difference—that makes you, you. But really, the self isn't just one thing.

Self is all of you.

Self is multitudes.

Self is everything.

*Whitman much?*

Google's definition notes something very interesting as well—that the self is especially defined by its status as an object of thought.

So it's as if the self only exists because you think about it existing.

You think about your sense of self, so therefore you have a sense of self.

*Descartes much?*

If it were enough to simply think your sense of self into existence, however, everyone would walk around confident, all mojo-ed up, making the universe awesome every single day.

What percentage of us does that?

Instead, it seems the self works in phases—awesome phases where we know just who we are and where we belong, followed by phases of uncertainty and questioning, followed by perhaps phases where we're not sure whether the self we once recognized ever truly existed.

That third phase doesn't just happen overnight. Losing your sense of self is a problem that seems to creep up on you.

It takes a long time to come to the realization that your sense of self is missing—and it likely doesn't occur to you until after several weeks or even months of stress, personal crises, important life decisions, and the resulting mental fatigue.

Or maybe you never even had a sense of self. It might take a lifetime to come to that realization.

In either case, you can't just flaunt your inner Descartes and think that self back into existence.

(I realize I am stretching the applicability and context of Descartes' famous observation, but humor me.)

Instead, what seems to be more effective is actually the opposite:

Find yourself by focusing on anything other than yourself.

Get back to who you really are by forgetting about trying to get back to who you really are.

That may seem kind of like saying that you should put gas in your car by not putting gas in your car—it seems counter-intuitive and perhaps even impossible. Our gut instinct, after all, is to get to a goal through a series of steps designed to bring us to that goal. And we're often encouraged to break goals down into a system, a manageable series of steps or processes, to ensure that we get what we want in a proper manner.

But the self is different—it's elusive, it's intangible, though we know damn well when we have it, and it's slippery.

Self is everything and multitudes, remember? It's not just a single quality to which we can point a finger and say, "There! There it is! That's my self!"

Since it's all-encompassing, since it's multitudinous, we can't go looking for it the same way we'd look for a new dress. If the self is everything, then it's everywhere.

So looking for it, the way you'd look for an object, seems akin to looking for air.

It's impossible.

The self seems best found while focusing on another passionate pursuit—an activity, a hobby, an art form, a religious pursuit, a subject matter, or a career path.

For me it was fitness.

Every time I felt like I had the most mojo, the most drive, the most solid hold of myself, I was in the throes of a focused workout or pursuing a specific fitness accomplishment. And every time I felt like I had lost myself, spending all my time thinking about that lost self only made me feel more lost.

For me, there's only one way to find that self once it's gone:

Pursue something productive, and pursue it passionately.

Your self will reappear when you are utterly devoted to something else, when your focus is very much on everything but yourself.

When it happens, you will have no idea that your self is about to show its existence.

But you will be all the more able to appreciate its presence when it does.

## *37*

I once thought the hardest thing I ever did was quit smoking.

Yes, that was hard. I threw things at David on day one. I might have sworn at a class full of high-school students on day three. And then I had to relearn every single daily habit, from my morning coffee to driving home from work each day, in the context of my new non-smoker identity.

But the difficulty of having to quit smoking has been thoroughly trumped by several things in my life in the two years from 2012-2014:

1. Taking time away from teaching, the only career that I've ever known.

2. Gaining 40 pounds as a result of using food to soothe myself as I learned how to identify myself without the context of teaching.

The process behind doing both of these things was obviously more complicated than what I have stated above, but what is accurate is those were the toughest two years of my life so far.

What proved to be almost as tough, however, was giving myself the necessary tools and support to get my body back to where I wanted it to be—fitter and leaner.

The "necessary tools and support" this requires involved much of the typical things one might need to accomplish any kind of body recomposition—smart training plans, sustainable diet plans, supportive friends & family, minimized life stress, plenty of regular sleep. But I found that what makes me capable of succeeding at my goals of being leaner and fitter also involves my perception of myself—and I don't mean my perception of the self I want to be when I reach my goals.

I mean my perception of myself in a given moment. What I think of myself today affects the self I become tomorrow.

When I first came to terms with the overeating and binge eating issues I had developed, I tried, fruitlessly, to lose weight. I tried everything that had worked for me before—I had a coach to guide my workouts and nutrition (even personal trainers hire coaches), I had minimal life stress, I had the support of everyone I knew, and I continued to get 7-8 hours of sleep per night.

Invariably, despite the well-laid plans, I would get 2-3 weeks of consistency under my belt, then I'd find myself imploding—and usually "imploding" meant going off-plan and eating everything under the sun.

Or at least everything in the fridge.

I read more books about behavior change, binge eating, mindless eating, emotional eating, successful goal setting—whatever sounded like something I could use.

But no amount of reading, or getting back on my nutrition, could change what I think was really keeping me back:

I didn't think I was worthy of success.

After all, I had failed a bunch of times in the previous two years.

I spent a lot of my time feeling like a failure. Despite the fact that I was legitimately pursuing a passion—nutrition. Despite the fact that I was the busiest trainer in my gym after being there less than a year. Despite the fact that I was about to finish a Master's degree in less than two total years.

My lack of self-love wasn't just evident when I fell off the nutrition wagon; I was perpetuating the feeling that I was undeserving in a hundred subtle ways.

I avoided buying myself clothes—for work and for the gym—that fit the body I had right then. I avoided going back to the gym where I had once been a trainer—even though my body looked exactly the same as it did when I finished working there—because I hadn't "improved" yet. I avoided cleaning out my closets when new seasons approached because I didn't want to confront the fact that nothing I owned fit me anymore.

Note that most of these things involve being uncomfortable in my own body—something that weight training and fitness helped me get over a long time ago. And yet here it was, again, coming out in my everyday life, even as I continued to train and do the fitness-related things that I loved.

I had to try to get past this sticking point.

I bought myself a winter coat that fit. I had been wearing the only coat I had that still zipped adequately, but it wasn't very warm. In fact, I was often wearing David's coats at night when walking the dog.

I cleaned my closets and drawers, throwing away the things I didn't love, and packing away the things I did love so I could attempt to wear them again. I suddenly had several empty drawers and a few open closet shelves.

I filled those with clothes that I liked—both for work and gym—so I could feel good about where I was instead of fighting with images of where I used to be, or even worse, where I "should be."

And I focused my workouts around what I was capable of and what makes me awesome—my strength, my ability to push myself to do new and more difficult things, my dedication.

What's interesting about these changes are the effects they had on my other habits. I didn't just feel better walking down the street. I felt better when I ate. I was more consistent—and it wasn't because I was any closer to my goals. It was because loving myself in the present caused me to feel more in touch with myself in the future.

It was because, in the end, successful change must stem from self-care, not from self-hate.

There's no longer a chasm between the me of today and the me of tomorrow. We aren't two separate beings. I'm no longer trying to repair a faulty me and replace it with a better me.

There is no faulty me. Me today isn't any less me than the me from tomorrow, even if I am working to make the tomorrow me better than I am today.

We are both me, and we are both awesome.

## *38*

I hated my hands for years.

I kept my nails fairly long, and I wore numerous rings throughout my early 20s—three to four on each hand, including thumb rings—to try and change how they looked. I sometimes referred to my "sausage fingers" as a way to deflect attention away from the fact that I was uncomfortable with my short, squat hands. You know, self-deprecation as a means of pretending to have self-confidence?

What? That doesn't work for you?

It didn't work for me, either. And while I didn't spend hours of my days trying to think up ways to hide my hands, I never actually liked them.

Until I started lifting.

See, you have a choice when you start lifting more than casually and start genuinely picking up heavy things: either you can buy lifting gloves, or you can tell your hands to woman up.

I chose the latter, and the result is clear.

My hands don't get soaked, moisturized, filed, massaged or trimmed very often. They aren't soft. They aren't dainty. They aren't polished. And they aren't pampered.

Sometimes, these hands actually hurt. Sometimes it hurts to open them fully and stretch them out, and sometimes it hurts to make a super tight fist.

Sometimes, they ache even when they're not working hard. The calluses sometimes throb for a while after a workout. The blood blister under my middle finger, a new development, is tender to the touch. The holes I put in my hand, on several occasions, by ripping off calluses, hurt.

Everyday objects pass through these hands roughly at times, objects that would otherwise go unnoticed—the passage of the steering wheel along the calluses while driving, the edges of a condiment jar being opened for the first time, the fabric handles of a grocery bag packed high with heavy vegetables. Even the smooth black finish of brand new yoga pants is often marred by my jagged palms that snag on that smoothness at every touch.

These hands work hard. They work hard no matter what I do in the gym, and they have yet to give up when a weight is heavy—even if my chest, my back, my legs are ready to cave.

These hands work all day. They grasp heavy things, but they also cook, wash, steer, push, pull, sew, wring, toss, throw, grab, release, slap, swipe, open, and close.

They feel. They touch. They typed these words.

These days, I don't talk about "sausage fingers." These days, I wear just two or three rings. I often forget to put them on before I go out. These days, I keep my nails short; nails just get in the way of everything my hands need to do.

And boy, do these hands do a lot.

They've earned their stripes.

## *39*

I used to think I was the shit.

I didn't walk around with the words "I am the shit" floating in neon lights behind my eyes. I didn't even know I was the shit. I just felt good. All the time. About everything—in every situation.

That's not to say I never felt frustrated, angry, worried, helpless, or confused. But when I was the shit, I handled those things, and I handled them easily:

*Stress from grades being due for the quarter? No problem. Grades got done. And I still managed to bench press.*

In the odd case where the problem was long-lasting or not easily remedied, I still felt awesome:

*Worried about trying to get into a Master's program in Nutrition when I didn't have a science background? Whatever. I can take Chem I, Chem II, and Anatomy all online. With online labs. And ace them. While finishing my personal trainer certification. And bench pressing.*

Even given a long period of generalized, repetitive stress, like the above, which happened just as I was initiating a career change, I coped.

Because I was the shit.

I'm not entirely sure when I stopped being the shit, but I'm pretty sure it coincided with the start of my binge eating problems. I'm sure it was more of a slow decline from "the shit" status to something else. I certainly didn't wake up one morning and realize that I was suddenly no longer awesome. More likely, chinks in my shit armor started appearing bits at a time, slowly accumulating, until all the awesomeness that comes with being the shit was eroded.

Without the shit armor, I wasn't the same at handling myself:

*Bad workout? Feeling unmotivated? Time to wallow in self-loathing. Have a pity party. Maybe eat peanut butter.*

*Stress of teaching? Every day felt like a turn on an emotional torture wheel. Even if I was still bench pressing.*

Without the shit armor, I was no longer "the shit." I was just plain shit.

It doesn't matter to me, now, why I made the switch from the shit to plain shit. What's relevant to me now is how I became the shit to begin with and how I got back to being the shit today.

(Because I am. I'm the shit. Again.)

It's not about a definitive moment of suddenly becoming the shit. It's not like flipping a shit switch. It's about a series of circumstances, a group of qualities or events or facts, that contribute to building up that armor, that lead to the manifestation of "the shit" status.

Most of the circumstances that contributed to my former "the shit" status—and to my current "the shit" status— were fitness-related:

I was invested in every minute of just about every workout. I never thought about a long-term or distant goal while training; I never thought about what I was wearing to work the next day or what I was going to eat post-workout. I thought about the bar or weight I was trying to move right at that minute. And on the next rep, I did it again, trying to feel every last little piece of anatomy responsible for making that rep happen. Every muscle, every joint, every breath.

I was invested in every part of just about every day. When I wasn't training, I was busy. I taught my classes with gusto, trying new things whenever I could. When I wasn't teaching, I was putting all my creative energy into reading about nutrition, fitness, and health. When I wasn't reading, I was writing blog posts. And when I wasn't writing blog posts, I was thoroughly enjoying whatever "down" time I had, even if it was just 20 minutes to stretch and watch TV at the end of the day.

I was invested in every part of just about every food choice I made. I never felt like I would rather be eating any food other than the one I had chosen to eat at that moment. I genuinely looked forward to everything I ate, even during dieting phases, and I planned my meals to ensure that I was enjoying rather than dreading them. I ate slowly. I took twenty minutes to eat my morning oatmeal and twenty minutes to eat my peanut butter at night. Not because I wanted to make them last artificially, but because it felt good—it felt right—to really enjoy foods.

I could probably list twenty other similar qualities that I had at the time, but there's already a pattern emerging here ("I was invested…"), and it can be replicated regardless of who you are or what you love to do:

If you wish to be the shit, you must have a productive, constant outlet for both physical and mental energy.

You must have several activities at which to excel.

You must have a willingness to be truly in the moment at all times.

I could parse this list a bit more, add in some qualifying statement about being willing to fail, maybe address some higher level qualities like confidence or creativity. And I could probably spend time saying these things are attainable by anyone, anywhere, anytime, in any field.

But I think the ideas are most salient at their simplest:

If you've got something positive to put your energy into, if you do things you're good at and do them often, if you generally don't sit around doing nothing for too long, AND—and this is probably the most difficult thing—if you can genuinely focus all that energy into the now instead of focusing longingly on either the future or the past...

Well, then you're probably the shit.

Congrats.

Now go do something awesome.

## *40*

I have a long history of existential crises.

When I was a kid, I couldn't sleep at night. My mind raced. I read a lot before bed, just to try to keep my mind focused on something that might eventually lull me to sleep. My mom even took me to the doctor once to ask about my sleeping issues. I think I was eight or nine at the time. Those issues didn't subside at all during my older years. I had problems falling asleep quickly all the way through my 20s. It wasn't until I quit smoking and started working out a little in my late 20s that I suddenly found myself able to fall asleep within 20 minutes of my head hitting the pillow.

That struggle to relax into sleep at night seems symbolic of my default approach to life in the past:

*Go hard, all the time.*

On paper, that kind of energy and dedication sounds admirable.

But my inability to turn off my capacity for work caused all of the existential crises of my life.

My first crisis was after freshman year of college. I was on a full scholarship to an expensive local school. I had graduated with really high expectations from a local "honors" high school. My entire life had been spent overachieving in everything (except sports), and after a year of continuing to do the same in college, I was exhausted and burned out. All I wanted to do was take naps and write poetry.

So I dropped out of college.

I withdrew from my first semester of sophomore year sometime around October. It was a sudden decision but one that was gradually building for months. My parents were worried. What if I didn't go back? My mother had left college early, for similar reasons, and she didn't go back. Would I do the same?

I did all kinds of adult things that year while everyone else I knew went to classes. I got my own apartment. I adopted a cat. I bought a real car. I worked full-time in an office, and I wrote all the poetry I wanted.

And when the next school year rolled around, I felt rested and refreshed. I was ready to go back.

My second existential crisis happened from 2011 through 2014.

*Yes, it lasted three years.*

I had been teaching full-time since 2003, and by 2011, I was exhausted and burned out. Again. All I wanted to do was lift weights, write nutrition articles, and eat peanut butter.

So I left teaching for a while.

While I was gone, I finished a Nutrition degree. I worked as a personal trainer full-time, eventually quitting that for a gig as a health coach with a local insurance company. I took on a few fitness side jobs. And I ate an awful lot — so much that I gained 40 pounds.

But when the end of my two-year absence from teaching rolled around, I was ready to go back.

After both existential crises, I couldn't simply go back to the way I did things BEFORE the crisis. I had to change the problem—my inability to modulate my work capacity—so that I wouldn't burn out again.

In college, this change came naturally. I had become financially independent at age 20. I had been paying my own rent, bills, and living expenses for long enough that I was going to have to work full-time if I wanted to go to college AND live on my own. There were no parents paying my tuition or board, no family members who had started a college fund for me. Whatever I spent I had to earn, and the time commitment needed to work full-time and go to college kept me from the same "go hard, all the time" mentality I'd had before.

After college, I managed to work full-time while in grad school full-time, and then I did the same as I finished my teaching certificate and student teaching placements.

My first existential crisis wound up making me better. I had to learn to be something more than just a student.

I had to make similar adjustments for my return to teaching. I couldn't go back and fall into the same trap. I was still personal training in the evenings, after all, and I wanted time to devote to writing when I could. So I made a few rules for my reincarnation as a teacher:

- *No grading papers at home.*
- *No planning lessons at home.*
- *No extracurricular assignments.*
- *No staying after required hours.*

That last one might sound harsh—what if a kid needed me to stay after required hours for extra help?—but the goal was not to shirk any responsibilities or student needs. Rather, my goal was to do everything within school hours, including addressing student needs and extras as required, by being better in the classroom.

This forced me to become so much more efficient, and I found myself getting more work done during my 40-minute free periods than I ever did in the hour or two I used to "work" on school things at home. I found better systems for doing tasks that used to take much longer, and I found faster grading systems than what I'd been using before.

My second existential crisis forced me to become a better teacher. And learning to control the binge eating problem that accompanied the existential crisis made me a better trainer.

Both crises, however, made me realize just what a misnomer the term "existential crisis" is.

There is no "crisis" in realizing you need something in your life to change.

The crisis comes from NOT acknowledging that need, from staying stuck where you know you don't belong. Sure, it's difficult to change your life, and yes, sometimes life is unhappy while that change is happening. Sometimes the change takes three years. Sometimes you gain 40 pounds from the stress of it. And sometimes you end up in a place you never thought you would've when you envisioned the trajectory of your future.

But I would rather face temporary discomfort head-on than settle for long-term dissatisfaction.

And I'd rather quit—and relearn the right way to do things—than continue to be mediocre.

# *41*

Get comfortable being uncomfortable.

You've heard that saying before, right?

On the surface, this idea rings true.

If we want to change, we have to do things we don't normally do—we have to move outside our comfort zone, outside our normal habits, to create that change.

The thing is, it's not as simple as the cliché makes it out to be.

Change doesn't happen automatically because you moved outside your comfort zone, and it's not even necessary to move as far outside your comfort zone as this idea might suggest.

People who make big, drastic overnight changes to their lives—who step really far outside their comfort zones in one fell swoop—tend to fail.

Why?

Because comfort zones aren't just about our habits.

Our habits, our routines, are part of what we use to identify ourselves—we often lack the ability to see the "self" as a unified sum of our parts, and we often identify with our behaviors, even the negative or unsuccessful ones, instead.

We identify ourselves as couch potatoes, as failed dieters, or as people who just get by, and changing all of the behaviors tied to these identities creates discomfort not just because we have to acquire new habits but because we also have to acquire a new identity.

In short, when we change everything all at once, we don't recognize ourselves. And it's hard to behave in all these new ways without a strong sense of self to propel those changes.

Instead, then, of thinking of change as such a huge step outside our comfort zones, I prefer to think of change as a place tangential to our comfort zones. Right on the edge of your normal life, there's a sweet spot, the spot where you can broaden yourself in small, meaningful ways. It's not too far from where you are now, so when you get there, you can still recognize your normal self in what you're doing.

The place where change happens is still outside the comfort zone—you're never going to change in any measurable way without stepping outside that boundary. But you don't have to shoot from 0 to 60 immediately to see measurable change.

Consider what can happen if you shoot for a target just on the periphery of your comfort zone. Your likelihood of success increases because the change you are reaching for isn't a far stretch from your normal state of being. And once you've hit that initial target, you can shoot for a new one just on the periphery of your new comfort zone.

Again, success—you know, the part of change that makes you feel all warm and fuzzy and more likely to keep trucking?—will be likely because your new comfort zone is close to the change itself.

Every small change you make by stepping even slightly outside your comfort zone serves to expand your comfort zone itself.

This is how behavior changes can accumulate over time. By picking a series of goals that represent measurable change but are still close to your current habits, you can create a progression of changes over time.

And the beauty of it?

Because the goals are seemingly small and easy to achieve, you might not even notice you're changing.

Look, everyone knows someone who can set a very distant, seemingly impossible goal and get from here to there with little trouble.

That's what I did when I quit smoking.

I quit pretty much cold turkey, with very little use of nicotine replacement therapies, and I have never relapsed. That's great for me, but I would never encourage everyone to try this.

The thing is, I wasn't reaching far outside my comfort zone. In fact, I would argue I had a larger comfort zone to start. For me, quitting cold turkey was not a far cry from what I thought I could accomplish.

It was uncomfortable, yes, and it was a struggle.

But it was just outside the periphery of my normal behaviors.

And that proximity is what made me successful— it wasn't some kind of superhuman willpower, not some magic ability to do the impossible.

For me, it was close to possible.

So how can we apply this to ourselves?

A few tips:

- Set a small goal to start—this could be a step toward something more later on.
- Set a goal you can control—you can't control weight loss, for example, but you can control your eating habits, your exercise habits, your sleep habits, and those things later contribute to weight loss.
- Set a goal that's reasonable *for you*—and don't compare your goal to anyone else's because your comfort zone might be bigger or smaller than hers.
- Set a measurable goal—so you know when you've been successful.
- Set a new goal following all of these same guidelines once you reach the first goal—and then do it again and again and again.

And the next thing you know, you'll have gone from 0 to 60.

You'll just do it reasonably—and in a way that teaches you how to sustain change over time. Because no one wants to change temporarily.

And what's the point of reaching a long-term goal if you can't maintain it?

## *42*

We give our dog treats when she does what she's asked.

She goes out, pees right away, and comes right back in?

*Cookie.*

She stops barking at the kids walking by when I tell her to stop?

*Cookie.*

Given that this pattern of cookie-as-reward is common among dog owners, the following statement, on the surface, appears to be true for us humans:

Don't reward yourself with food. You're not a dog.

When I first started seeing this statement, or variations on it, going around Facebook and other social media, it seemed harmless.

After all, we aren't dogs, right?

*Right.*

Well, sort of.

The thing is, we actually are like dogs when it comes to learning new behaviors.

And that's not a bad thing.

But it's not the only thing wrong with this view of food rewards—in fact, I count four primary problems with the idea that humans shouldn't reward themselves with food:

1. Cookies aren't the only reward for dogs.

When I'm not near the dog cookies, and I ask my dog to do something, she still gets rewarded for listening to me. Instead of a cookie, however, she gets some token of affection—a good pat on the head, several "good dog" reassurances, sometimes a little belly rub.

In other words, equating food rewards with dog-hood is misleading. Dogs aren't only motivated by food (though some are more than others), and just like dogs, people aren't only motivated by food (though some are more than others).

So to equate food rewards with being a dog is, simply, a gross oversimplification.

Different dogs respond to different motivations. So do different people.

## 2. Not all food rewards are negative: Part 1

The statement, "Don't reward yourself with food. You're not a dog," implies that the food used in the reward is bad.

What makes a food "bad"?

I would argue no foods are "bad" and that there are only healthy and unhealthy choices. And even then, foods we might consider to be "healthy" can be unhealthy in large amounts, and foods we might consider to be "unhealthy" can be fine in moderate amounts.

But let's assume the statement is intended to keep people from rewarding themselves with generally unhealthy food choices—traditional "reward" foods like cakes, cookies, sweets, and other high-calorie, indulgent options.

We've all experienced food used in this way—even having indulgent, special food on a special occasion is a reward of sorts.

You got a job promotion? Let's celebrate with pizza!

You made it to the big 40? Here's a big old cake!

We already use food as a reward in our culture—and that's not a bad thing. It's not bad to go out for a special dinner to celebrate a job promotion. It's not bad to have cake on your birthday.

We even use food in this way with our dogs.

My dog doesn't know why she's getting a giant doggy cupcake on her birthday. She doesn't know why I gave her roasted turkey on Thanksgiving. She probably just thinks she's lucky.

Our sense of celebration—and reward—is intrinsically human, not canine.

Calling all food rewards bad is, again, an oversimplification.

And it denies us something unique to humans—our ability to honor the awesome in each other.

3. Not all food rewards are negative: Part 2

When we think of food as a reward, we think of treat foods. We've already established this.

But why?

Isn't it a reward to feed ourselves after a hard workout? And is it less of a reward if I choose to feed myself healthy foods? I look forward to post-workout meals— and it isn't because I'm hungry. Frankly, working out temporarily kills my appetite.

Instead, I love eating post-workout because I know I am helping my body recover. The protein, the carbs—my body needs it all after a workout to get stronger, repair itself, and prepare for the next workout.

At first, when I thought of this objection to the idea that only dogs get food as a reward, I thought maybe this only applied to me.

But I don't think so.

I see evidence of this in almost everyone I know who works out hard. We genuinely look forward to food. It feels satisfying—and therefore rewarding—to feed ourselves healthy food, especially after a workout.

That's not to say there aren't unhealthy examples of this, such as in those with eating disorders, where the reward of a post-workout meal might be the only meal in a day.

But in an otherwise healthy, fit person, even healthy food can be a reward.

4. We need rewards to function. Like NEEEED them.

One of the best books I've read was *The Power of Habit* by Charles Duhigg.

The most important thing I learned from that book was actually quite simple—the habit loop. We need a series of specific things to build a habit. We need a cue, or some kind of trigger, a routine, or some path of behavior to enact, and a reward.

That's right—we need rewards to build habits.

This works negatively, like the reward of a nicotine buzz at the end of a cigarette smoking habit loop. But it also works positively, like the reward of an endorphin rush from intense exercise.

In the book, Duhigg talks about changing a simple unhealthy habit—eating a cookie every afternoon at work—to a healthy one. The process involved recognizing the cue or trigger (for him, this was the time, say 3:30 every day), recognizing the routine that ensued from the cue (walking to the cafeteria to get said cookie), and recognizing the reward (a break from work, a sugar rush, and a little socializing in the cafeteria with friends).

To change this habit loop, he first considered what reward he was seeking with his behavior. Was he hungry? Or just looking for some socialization and a break from work?

Ultimately, he decided it was the latter. To change his routine, then, he kept the trigger the same (3:30 every day), changed the routine, and kept the reward similar. Instead of the quest for a cookie, his new routine was to seek out a co-worker—giving him the same socialization reward he originally sought.

This is how I've started helping clients and coaching patients create new behaviors. We identify the cue for a behavior, identify the routine that person goes through, and identify the reward. We keep the cue and the reward the same, change the routine, and the person gets a new healthy version of an old habit.

This isn't, of course, foolproof; stress often knocks people off even their most well-intentioned new habits, and old behaviors start to creep back into their lives instead. But knowing that there still needs to be a reward—as in, you must enjoy something about your new habits—makes creating new behaviors that much easier.

And it flies in the face of the idea that rewards are just for dogs.

Because really, aren't we using a habit loop with our dogs, too?

Cue? Tell her to sit. Routine? She puts her butt on the floor. Reward? Cookie or "good girl."

Human habit loops aren't so different than dog habit loops.

And our need for rewards isn't all that different, either.

So reward yourself. You aren't a dog if you do so.

In fact, you're quite human.

## *43*

I played the flute as a kid.

I'm not sure how I chose flute over the saxophone, which I vaguely remember wishing I could play. Yet I played the flute from 5th through 12th grade, and I was in and out of my high school marching band and concert band throughout those years.

Somewhere in those band years, I also poorly played the oboe. Double reeds are difficult, yo.

At some point, I also learned piano, and later I was gifted an acoustic guitar, on which I did nothing but practice "Edelweiss." I eventually broke one of the tuning pegs in a poor attempt at tuning.

Despite knowing, on paper, how to "play" these instruments, I never became very good at a single one of them, though I was proficient at flute. The problem wasn't knowledge. I knew my music theory, I knew my sight reading, and I knew my fingering.

The problem was how I practiced: I only did so moderately.

I didn't apply any of my normal work ethic to my musical instruments. I gave flute more hard work than anything else, but even then, I gave flute less time than I gave singing, or calculus, or poetry. So by the end of high school, while I had some musical skills, what was I really good at? Singing. Calculus. And poetry.

The things we become well-versed in are the things on which we spend the most energy, and the things at which we are just average are the things on which we spend average energy. My moderate practice habits—not too much, not too little—made me a mediocre musician.

If you've read Malcolm Gladwell's *Outliers*, you probably recognize something of his 10,000-hour rule in this.

The 10,000-hour rule suggests "experts" with a talent for something specific spend at least 10,000 hours perfecting those skills. Gladwell shows that for many "experts," getting to spend that kind of excessive time honing a skill is partly a matter of luck—being born in the right era, with access to the right education, or the right people, with the right social skills.

Luck + excessive time = greatness.

Notice that moderation isn't part of that equation.

If we define "moderation" as restraint from excesses—if moderation is about doing not too much but not too little—then becoming good at something means avoiding moderation. And that applies to anything we wish to become good at, including our ability to lose weight.

Despite the popularity of branded diet programs, the very simple "everything in moderation" mantra is itself a popular weight loss plan. I've had scores of clients choose NOT to have me help them with diet in favor of trying moderation as a plan instead.

And I'm not exaggerating when I say 100% of my clients that used moderation as a weight loss plan struggled to lose weight.

The problem is not with the idea that you can eat a little of everything and still lose weight. The problem is "everything in moderation" gives you the illusion that weight loss isn't a skill, that it doesn't need to be planned, and that it's not something you have to repeatedly work at, with effort, to see results.

And weight loss is a skill. It's just a skill many have yet to master. Plus, more likely than not, you have an opposing skill—overeating, or maybe, like me, binge eating—at which you have become a genuine expert. And the 10,000 hours you've spent honing your overeating or binge eating skills will take planning and repeated effort, not moderation, to overcome.

I know you're going to protest by showing me a picture of your friend, or trainer, who practices moderation and maintains her jacked and tan physique by doing so.

But listen:

She didn't get jacked and tan without putting in her figurative 10,000 hours. Moderation is a great way to maintain your expert skills. But if you're not a pro, you have to put in the time before you can get there.

## *44*

I have only lived one biological life. And it has been rife with existential crises.

But I have found myself reborn multiple times: once, at 19, when I dropped out of college. Again, at 20, when I returned to college as an English major; yet again, at 25, when, after pursuing entrance to a Ph.D. program, I ultimately decided to pursue teaching high school. A fourth time at 30 when I was struggling to make ends meet for four years on a private school salary. Then, there was age 32, when I started lifting weights and realized the capabilities of my physical body. Once more, at 35, when I realized I needed to step away from teaching to pursue other interests.

Somewhere within all those reincarnations, I called myself a poet, a bookkeeper, a vegetarian, an omnivore, a scholar, a grad student, a fiction writer, an essayist, a blogger, a cook, a student, a personal trainer, a coach, a health coach, and a philosopher.

In the Spring of 2014, I decided to undergo yet another reincarnation, this time in a role with which I was already very familiar:

As a teacher.

In April, I decided to return to my position as a high school English teacher for the 2014-2015 school year.

I subsequently resigned from my position with a local health insurance company, where I had been working as a health coach for the previous year.

Like every reincarnation I have been through, I was excited and nervous to make this transition.

The work I was doing as a health coach wasn't a bad gig. Many of my post-binge eating blog posts were born from my work in behavior change and health coaching. Health coaching was work that made me feel like I was doing something good—like I was helping people who needed the help.

But something was pulling at my commitment to that health coaching work for a while, and teaching was always in the back of my mind. It wasn't that I was constantly thinking about going back to teaching, though I found myself consciously considering that question more every day.

What pulled me back into teaching was something more intangible, something I couldn't really put into words.

Until I was sitting at my desk in my office downtown one Friday, and I turned to my left to see an old newspaper clipping on my pegboard. It was a My View editorial honoring Mr. Soffin, my high school Math teacher, and it had been written by Mr. Duggan, my high school English teacher.

I had that newspaper clipping for years and still do. It hung next to my desk at the private school where I taught for the first four years of my career. It hung next to my desk at the public school where I taught for the next five years. It even followed me to my desk at the insurance company.

So the idea of teaching—even when I wasn't a teacher—literally never left my side.

That Friday, when I turned to my left and reread that newspaper clipping for what seemed like the millionth time, I knew why I hadn't been able to articulate my thoughts about teaching, even though I thought about it every day.

I was afraid that articulating something definitive about it, and returning to it, meant that I was moving backward, rather than forward, in some way.

Don't mistake what I mean by this—I do not mean that taking time away from teaching was a mistake.

It wasn't.

But going back is hard. And there were things about teaching that I was struggling with, terribly, when I left. I felt like I was investing so much of myself—my time, my energy, my emotional capacity—to my teaching that I couldn't invest myself in other areas of my life.

And I am most certainly the kind of person who invests herself in everything she does. It isn't worth doing, in my mind, if I cannot do it wholeheartedly.

That devotion to what I do most certainly played into my decision to leave teaching as well—leaving was the hardest decision I ever made.

But I recognized, after rereading that newspaper clipping, I had unfinished business as a teacher, unfinished business that trumped my fear of returning. And that business wasn't with students, or colleagues, or administrators, or even the literature I would be teaching.

No, that unfinished business was with me.

My identity, for the last ten years, had been wrapped up in the word "teacher" in every way possible. I taught students, yes, but I also found my teacher identity was one that leaked into everything else I did.

As a blogger, as a trainer, as a coach, even as a partner, I am, at my core, a teacher.

Not being a teacher for the last two years had left me with an odd sense of identity—it was no secret, nor a coincidence, that my struggle with food and weight happened concurrently with my decision to leave teaching.

So the decision to go back to teaching, despite all my resistance to even thinking about it, turned out to be the easiest one I've ever made.

Because teaching is who I am.

And knowing that is both a relief and a rebirth.

It made me, me again.

No matter how many other "lives" I have lived, no matter what I called myself during those lives—poet, coach, trainer, or otherwise—they all fall under the only name that matters:

Me, Kristen, the teacher.

That's a name, and a rebirth, worth living.

## *45*

I always loved hearing from my blog's readers. I once got an email from someone trying to get back into some healthy food & fitness habits.

After emailing her with some very basic workout and food suggestions, I started thinking about what I would tell *anyone* just starting a new fitness or nutrition program.

I could go beyond these seven tips, but I think these are very smart, honest, and useful starting points:

1. Do it for the right reasons.

How many times have you heard someone say she was going to start working out to get ready for her wedding? Or a vacation? Or so she'd look good for a reunion?

Or how about the girl who runs 3 miles every day to justify eating junk foods?

There's nothing wrong with admitting that part of our reason for training is to look a certain way. By saying I'm into bodybuilding, I am admitting my focus on aesthetics upfront.

But aesthetics are not what will keep most people in the gym in the long run. In fact, any reason that doesn't involve long-term goals is probably not a motivator for lifelong fitness.

If you are going to embark on a new fitness program, your reasons should be ones that will sustain your decision for some time to come. This might include:

- maintaining health and longevity
- becoming stronger
- gaining energy and endurance
- strengthening bones to prevent osteoporosis
- preventing or correcting medical conditions like heart disease, high blood pressure, diabetes, or high cholesterol
- preventing or correcting physical performance issues like posture problems, joint weaknesses, muscle imbalances, or previous injuries
- setting a good example for the rest of your family, including children
- and finally, improving mood and ability to cope with stress

Just like anything else, if you are doing it for superficial reasons, you're likely to fail.

Embark on a new fitness program because you want the good stuff—the life-affirming and life-prolonging stuff—and I guarantee you'll end up looking good anyway.

2. Keep a food journal.


This doesn't have to be permanent, but for at least a
while, I think any new fitness devotee needs to make
herself aware of her own food intake.


The best way to do this is to write everything down:


- time of meal
- foods eaten
- amounts of food eaten
- additional thoughts while eating (i.e., mood,
  whether you were genuinely hungry, bored, etc.)


Not everyone needs to do what I did—nerdy spreadsheets
tracking macros are not a good idea for everyone. But a
simple sheet of paper (or several) keeping track of food
will give you a strong idea of exactly what you're eating
and how much of it you eat in a day.


It will give you insight into areas where you can improve
your choices, add healthy veggies and fruits, cut
quantities, or swap foods. It will also help you figure out
what works well for your body and your workouts once
you begin a fitness program.


3. Measure your progress by comparing yourself to
yourself.

It's great to have fitness aspirations and role models to which you look for motivation. I have lots of them—and I look to them and their dedication for continued drive and focus when I sometimes fall short on my own.

But you should never, ever determine your own success or failure by comparing your results to someone else.

The fact is your body doesn't understand the difference between the number of push-ups you can do versus the number of push-ups the girl next to you can do. All your body knows is how hard it has worked—it knows if you're pushing it to its full capacity, and it knows when you're easy on it.

As long as you are always pushing your body as hard as you can, you will progress. You will change. Your body will get stronger and better and faster and smarter.

Your progress should be measured by how far you've come, not by unrealistically comparing your ability or your body to another's.

And if you have seen genuine progress, if you can genuinely do more, go faster, or lift heavier, then you should consider yourself successful. Because you are.

4. Be consistent.

I was sort of a jack-of-all-trades when it came to music-related activities in high school. I played the flute, I dabbled in the oboe, and I sang in 2 choruses. I was in musicals and concert band. I lived music.

And then college came along, and I half-heartedly went to choral practices and let my flute collect dust.

Today, I sing the way everyone else does—loudly, badly, in my car or the shower—when no one else is listening. And it's not because I've lost whatever minuscule innate talent I had as a kid.

It's because I was inconsistent.

I didn't practice. I let my fingers forget the flute scales. I let my voice lose its extended range.

In short, I didn't keep it up.

The same goes for fitness and nutrition. One day of cardio will not change you. One day of healthy eating will not change you.

One week of training will not change you, and one full week of healthy food will not change you either. Results—good ones, long-term ones, the kind you can be proud of—take time.

Give yourself time, and honor your commitment by being consistent in those efforts.

5. Learn how to make 3-4 healthy meals that you genuinely love.

I am very annoyed by and tired of hearing people say that healthy food doesn't "taste" good. If you made it, and it sucks, figure out how to make it better.

It takes 2-3 weeks of consistency to grow accustomed to new tastes and new foods. See #4 above.

But aside from this, healthy doesn't need to mean bland, nor does it need to mean boring and plain.

Buy a cookbook. Read an *Eating Well* magazine. Or *Cooking Light.* Google recipes.

Most importantly, cook things. Often.

And then, when you've found a few healthy things you enjoy making and eating, keep making them. Savor them. Look forward to them.

Then repeat this daily.

6. The worst, most stressful days are probably the best days to train.

Maybe this seems counterintuitive, but in my experience, the days when I am most stressed, most annoyed, or most frazzled are the best days to workout.

You won't necessarily have the greatest workout on these days. If your head's not there, you might lack the focus required for the best training session ever.

But the best way to fail at a goal is to let outside problems—things that have nothing to do with your fitness goals—get in the way of achieving what you want.

Annoying co-workers? Train anyway.

Boss in a tizzy? Train anyway.

Customers in your face? Train anyway.

Yes, there are genuinely stressful life events that might prevent getting in a scheduled workout. Sickness, injury, tragedy, and emergencies happen to all of us.

But letting the occasional bad day get the best of your fitness plans starts you on a slippery slope of habitually missing workouts. And you're bound to try to de-stress in other ways, some of which may be unhealthy.

Let the bad days be the reason to get it done, not the excuse to skip out.

7. Start today.

Are you waiting for January 1st? To make a resolution?

Are you waiting until after someone's party, birthday, dinner, or luncheon?

People who wait are most likely to fail in the long run. What's wrong with starting tomorrow? Is there something holding you back, something you think will prevent your fresh start?

Then be honest: you don't really want it.

Example: I intended to quit smoking for years.

For many years—probably for 8 of the ten years during which I smoked a pack of cigarettes a day—I really, in my head, wanted to quit.

But I didn't.

When I truly wanted it, however, when I had truly decided it was time to make that change, I quit that morning.

On Saturday, February 26, 2005, I woke up, went to Rite-Aid, bought some Nicorette, and haven't smoked since.

I didn't wait for an arbitrary date like New Year's Day. I didn't wait until AFTER the next big night out or the next big stressful week.

I wanted it, so I did it.

If you want it, start today.

Not tomorrow.

Now.

# *Afterword*

In November of 2016, I wrote my last *Following Fit* post.

I didn't know it would be my last.

By then, I was focusing the website on training articles, emphasizing my role as a coach, as an expert, rather than focusing on my reflections about who I was or where I'd been. I spent 2015 and 2016 writing about how to meal prep, about how to choose the right foods for a fat loss diet, about how to train around a busted SI joint—about everything except myself. I was training clients again, in the evenings and remotely, and I wanted *Following Fit* to support that side business.

But my heart wasn't in that writing.

After I wrote what became the last *Following Fit* post, I told myself I would let *Following Fit* die if I had nothing to say there in the next year. November 2017 came and went, and I wrote nothing on *Following Fit*. My training business grew, despite my lack of publishing, and half of 2018 flew by before I decided it was time to let *Following Fit* go.

The decision to end *Following Fit* was not an easy one. *Following Fit* was where I became me, as a trainee, as a trainer, as a nutrition coach, and as a recovering binge eater. It was also where I found my voice as a writer, and in 2018, I knew I no longer wanted to be restricted to fitness and nutrition topics.

I no longer wanted to be a fitness writer.

I just wanted to be a writer.

Despite having been the place where I became the me I was, *Following Fit* was no longer a suitable place for the me to come. And so I did what I have always done—I cut my ties with that which was keeping me from growing, and I let myself change.

In June, I started the process of shutting *Following Fit* down. I extracted all the posts so I could keep them. I changed my social media profiles to reflect my name instead of my brand name. I started a new website, with no fitness branding, so that I could publish essays, stories, poems—anything I wanted—without being beholden to a subject matter.

One day, someone asked me about my reasons for ending *Following Fit*. I told her the truth—*Following Fit* just wasn't a complete picture of me anymore. It was time to move on.

"You're so brave," she said.

It struck me as odd, the idea that it was brave to admit it was time to move on, because moving on to new things has always just been a thing I do. It was time, for example, when I was 27, to quit smoking. It was time, when I was 32, to lift weights and get strong. It was time, when I was 35, to consider a career change, and it was time, when I was 41, to get married despite thinking I never would.

I never saw it as brave to change. I just changed.

That willingness to change is the best underlying message *Following Fit* has left with me. It doesn't matter if I was vegetarian and then wasn't; it doesn't matter if I was lean as fuck and then wasn't.

What matters is the flexibility to become something new when the time was right. I found that flexibility through fitness, but it has changed my teaching, my relationships, and my writing. That's the magic of fitness. It isn't only about the body.

Fitness grew, for me, like the limbs of a tree, and while my newest branches and leaves might be far from the trunk where I started, all my new growth feeds on that trunk, and that trunk feeds on the roots below that.

They are all me, future, past, and present—multitudes connected in one living, breathing, changing self.

# *Acknowledgments*

When I joined a gym for the first time in 2009, I got a few free training sessions as part of my membership. I was assigned to a trainer, and we played phone tag a few times, trying to schedule a time to meet. After a few attempts, however, that trainer stopped returning my calls, and I found myself at the gym's front desk, asking if I could use my sessions with someone else. The guy at the desk said sure—how about using them with him?

The guy at that desk was Chris Rombola, and not only did I train with Chris then, but I have continued to train with him ever since. In March of 2011, during one of my training sessions, he taught me how to pose like a bodybuilder, taking pictures for me on my phone. One of those pictures became the central image on *Following Fit*, and that picture is now the cover of this book. Chris has since been my coach, my friend, my marriage officiant, and my mentor, and his guidance as I dove head first into fitness has been invaluable.

I would never hear the end of it if I didn't also acknowledge my brother, Todd Perillo, with whom I joined that first gym back in 2009. We went into fitness together, later saw our fitness paths diverge as I engulfed myself in the field, and then celebrated as those paths came together last year when Todd became one of my personal training clients. The truth is that I would be thanking Todd here regardless of our gym exploits together in 2009 and regardless of any brotherly teasing I might receive if I left him out. His support has always been unwavering, and his friendship extends beyond gym walls.

In the years that I was blogging at *Following Fit*, I had a network of support that I never imagined would develop from my little website. I had teaching colleagues, like Danielle Diina, who became fitness buddies and who gave me insightful feedback on everything I wrote. I had blogging colleagues, too, whose comments on my writing and private messages helped me see fitness in ways I hadn't yet. Juliet Gentile was the first person to read my binge eating confession, and her support and insistence that I had to make that story public gave me the courage to hit publish that day. Later, when I wished to turn this into a book, I had Peter Baker serve as my editor. I've actually never met Peter, but I knew from my online interactions with him that he was real, he was honest, and he would tell me what I needed to hear.

My husband, David, of course, also needs thanks. David has never had a lot to say about my passion for fitness and nutrition, but that is precisely the kind of support I need from him. David gives me the space to do the things I need to do, even when those things are separate from him, and our connection has grown stronger even as we have both grown differently over the last 17 years. I've watched many people suffer through relationship turmoil when fitness became a personal priority; as their bodies changed, so did their relationships, sometimes for the worse. David has accepted both me and my body in all of their incarnations. Whether I have been lean and shredded, heavy from binging, or muscular and athletic; whether I have been a teacher, a trainer, a nutritionist, or a writer, David has welcomed all of them, all of me, with no questions.

Lastly, there are the other women in my very first gym, the ones I looked up to when I was squatting a twelve-pound body bar and struggling to run laps around the building in boot camp. Those women, so much fitter than I was, were doing things I never thought I could, and their work ethic made me want to do the same. I wanted to be them, and I pushed myself just a little harder any time I lagged too far behind them. Within a few years, I accumulated my own list of personal bests, fitness feats I was proud I had accomplished, and I no longer compared myself to them. Whether they knew it or not, those women allowed me to stand on their strong shoulders. As more and more women turn to fitness and strength training, they, too, will look to the women around them in the gym for guidance, and I hope that they will look to me. It's my job to make sure that my shoulders are strong enough to bear that burden—a burden that's not a hardship, not an encumbrance, but a privilege and a genuine honor.

Made in the USA
Middletown, DE
20 December 2018